Guest Check

PERSONS	SERVER	TABLE	CHECK
1	V.C.	4	01240

nibbles and bites

Healthy And Elegant Appetizer Recipes For Entertaining

Valerie Reneé Campbell

Copyright © 2011 by Valerie Renee' Campbell

All rights reserved. No part of this publication may be reproduced,
in any manner, without the prior written permission of the publisher.

Published by
Empower Publishing
New York, New York 10023

Design by
Lucien Liz-Lepiorz

Library of Congress Catalog Number: 2009943582

ISBN: 0-9761760-3-3
ISBN 13: 978-0-9761760-3-9

Printed in the United States of America

In memory of my father and grandfather,

Command Sergeant Major Lacy McDougald, Jr.
November 6, 1934 - May 12, 2000

Robert Hill Terry, Sr.
August 29, 1928 - August 23, 2003

To my loving mother, Barbara McDougald; my grandmother, Jessie Terry; my sisters, Terry and Jessica; my nephews and nieces, Tyler, Bria, Justyn and Kristian; my brothers-in-law, Will and Alonzo; my family and friends, my awesome surgeon, Terrence M. Fullum, M.D.; my wonderful PCP, Dr. Paul Barone, and my Facebook fans.

Thanks for your continued support of my works.

CONTENTS

Veggies & Fruit Appetizers	2
Cold Finger Foods	21
Hot Finger Foods	28
Fowl Treats	35
Beef Treats	40
Seafood Fare	49
Asian Influences	60
Meatless Party Solutions	68
Sweet Treats	77
Drinks & Shooters	82

care for something to start with?

VEGGIES & FRUIT APPETIZERS

Jazzed Up Olives

Makes 12 servings

Ingredients:
- 1 1/2 cups green and black olives - drained
- 1 clove garlic - minced
- 4 tablespoons extra virgin olive oil
- 1/2 teaspoon red pepper flakes
- 1 lemon
- Fresh ground pepper (to taste)

Directions:

- Combine olives, garlic, oil, and pepper flakes in a large sealable plastic bag.
- Zest one lemon and add the lemon zest to the olive mixture and add ground black pepper.
- Let olives sit at room temperature for at least 2-3 hours.

May be refrigerated for up to 3 days. Allow to sit till room temperature before serving.

Warm Black Olives

Makes 8 to 10 servings

Ingredients:
- 1 pound large black olives
- 3 tablespoons extra virgin olive oil
- 4 slices prosciutto - torn into tiny pieces
- 8 fresh sage leaves
- 4 bay leaves
- 2 African bird's eye chiles or habanera chiles
- 1 tablespoon sea salt or lite salt

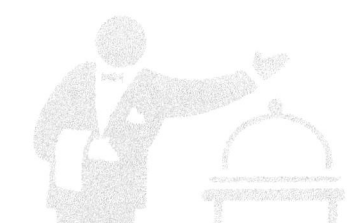

Directions:
- Drain olives, rinse, and oil pat dry.
- Heat olive oil in a pan over medium heat.
- Add olives and fry. Stir constantly for about 2-3 minutes.
- Add prosciutto, chiles, sage, and bay leaves and lightly toss. Add salt and remove from heat. Stir lightly.
- Transfer to a serving bowl and serve warm.

Mushroom Appetizers

Makes 8 servings

Ingredients:
- 16 ounces package of whole fresh mushrooms (Do not use canned)
- 8 ounces bottle vinaigrette salad dressing
- 1/2 large sweet onion sliced in wedges with layers separated

Directions:
- Rinse and place mushrooms in a container that can be tightly sealed.
- Trim any hard stems if necessary. Add onion to the container.
- Coat mushrooms with dressing.
- Seal and refrigerate for 3 hours.
- Occasionally shake the container.
- Serve as an appetizer or snack on a relish tray and drizzle dressing over the mushrooms to keep them moist. Or serve on skewers with black and green olives and cubes of hard cheeses on trays.

Marinated Mushrooms & Artichokes

Makes 10 servings

Ingredients:
- 1/2 cup Vinegar
- 1/2 cup Olive oil
- 2 cloves garlic - minced
- 2 tablespoons Water
- 2 teaspoons Granulated sugar
- Lite salt (to taste)
- 1 teaspoon dried basil and thyme
- 1 pound Small mushrooms
- 1 can Artichoke pieces in water - drained
- Italian parsley
- Cherry tomatoes
- Black olives

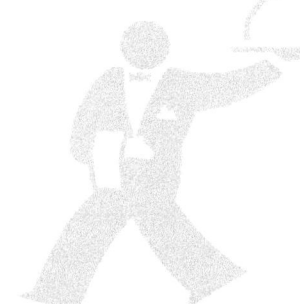

Directions:
- In large mixing bowl, whisk together vinegar, oil, garlic, water, sugar, basil and thyme. Add mushrooms and artichokes; stir to mix. Cover and refrigerate for at least 1 day or up to 10 days, stirring occasionally.
- Before serving, drain vegetables. Garnish with Italian parsley, cherry tomatoes and black olives (if using). Serve with cocktail picks.

Lime & Honey Pears

Makes 4 servings

Ingredients:
- 1/2 cup honey
- 1/4 cup water
- 1/4 cup lime juice
- 1/2 teaspoon grated lime peel
- 2 firm, ripe pears - cored, halved, pared

Directions:
- To microwave: Combine honey, water and lime juice in 2-quart microwave-safe dish; microwave at HIGH (100%) 2-1/2 to 3 minutes or until mixture boils.
- Stir in lime peel. Add pear halves to syrup; cover with vented plastic wrap and microwave at HIGH 7 to 10 minutes or until pears are tender.
- Serve warm or cold with poaching liquid.

Fig Appetizers with Goat Cheese and Almonds

Ingredients:
- 12 fresh figs - halved
- 4 ounces herbed goat cheese (chevre)
- 24 almonds
- 1 tablespoon honey
- 2 teaspoons balsamic vinegar

Directions:
- Preheat the oven broiler for high heat.
- Place the fig halves, cut side up, on a baking sheet. Top each half with about 1/2 teaspoon goat cheese. Place one almond on each, press to push the cheese slightly into each fig.
- Broil the figs in the preheated oven until the cheese is soft and the almonds are turning a rich shade of brown, 2 to 3 minutes. Remove from the broiler and let cool for 5 minutes. Arrange the figs on a serving platter and drizzle with honey and balsamic vinegar. Serve warm.
- Arrange figs in a circle, tops facing in, for a flower effect.

Grape and Avocado Salsa

Ingredients:
- 1 1/2 cups seedless red grapes - chopped
- 1 avocado - peeled, pitted and diced
- 1/4 cup chopped red bell pepper
- 2 tablespoons chopped yellow bell pepper
- 2 tablespoons chopped sweet onion

- 2 tablespoons chopped fresh cilantro
- 1 tablespoon lime juice
- 1/2 teaspoon garlic salt
- 1 pinch ground black pepper

Directions:
- Place the grapes, avocado, red pepper, yellow pepper, onion, and cilantro in a mixing bowl. Season with lime juice, garlic salt, and black pepper. Gently fold the ingredients together until well mixed. Refrigerate 30 minutes before serving.

Avocado Mango Salsa

Ingredients:
- 1 avocado - peeled, pitted and diced
- 1 lime, juiced
- 1 mango - peeled, seeded and diced
- 1 small red onion, chopped
- 1 habanero pepper, seeded and chopped
- 1 tablespoon chopped fresh cilantro
- Salt (to taste)

Directions:
- Place the avocado in a serving bowl, and mix with the lime juice. Mix in the mango, onion, habanero pepper, cilantro and salt. Note: Always wear gloves when handling habanero peppers.

Brazilian Onion Bites

Makes 12 servings

Ingredients:
- 1 small sweet onion - peeled
- 6 tablespoons mayonnaise
- Kosher salt (to taste)
- Freshly ground black pepper (to taste)
- 6 thin slices white bread - crusts removed
- 4 tablespoons freshly grated Parmesan cheese

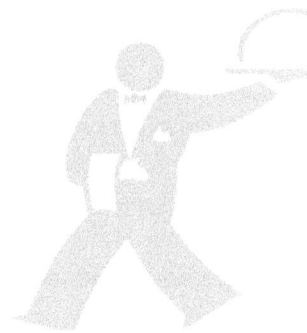

Directions:
- Preheat the oven to 350° F.
- Quarter onion lengthwise, then cut into thin slivers crosswise.
- Mix the onion with 5 tablespoons of the mayonnaise and salt and pepper to taste. Set aside.
- Spread 3 slices of bread on one side with the remaining mayonnaise.

(continued)
- Cut these into quarters.

- Cut the remaining 3 slices of bread into quarters and spread each square evenly with the onion mixture.
- Top with the reserved bread squares, mayonnaise side up.
- Place these on a baking sheet and sprinkle the tops generously with Parmesan cheese.
- Bake until lightly golden and slightly puffy, about 15 minutes. Serve immediately.

French Onion Quiche Appetizers

Makes 30 pieces

Ingredients:
- 1 package (15 ounce size) refrigerated pie crust dough

Filling:
- 1/4 cup margarine or butter
- 1 1/2 cup finely chopped onions
- 1 tablespoon flour
- 1 cup half and half
- 3 eggs, slightly beaten
- 1/2 teaspoon lite salt
- 1/8 teaspoon pepper
- 5 tablespoons grated Parmesan cheese

Directions:
- Heat oven to 350° F. Remove pie crust pouches from box. Let stand at room temperature 15 to 20 minutes while preparing filling.
- In medium pan, melt margarine; saute onion until light gold brown. Remove from heat. Stir in flour. Add half land half, eggs, salt land pepper. blend well.
- Unfold pie crusts; peel off plastic sheets. Press out fold lines. With floured 2 1/2" cookie. cutter, cut 15 circles from each pie crust sheet.
- Press each circle into ungreased miniature muffin cups. Spoon about 1 Tablespoon filling into each crust. Sprinkle each with 1/2 teaspoon cheese. Bake at 350F for 25 to 35 minutes or until centers are set and crusts are light golden brown.
- If filling becomes too brown, cover with foil last 10 minutes. Cool slightly. Remove from muffin cups. Serve warm.

Onion Bhaji

Makes 4 servings

Ingredients:
- 2 onions
- 1/2 teaspoon cumin, ground

- 1 egg - beaten
- 1 pinch cayenne pepper
- 1 1/2 cup chick pea flour (besan)
- 2 tablespoons fresh cilantro, chopped
- 1 cup cold water, approximately

Directions:
- Cut the onion in half and slice it about 1/4 inch thick. Beat together egg, flour and enough water to make a batter as thick as whipping cream. Beat in spices. Let rest 15 minutes. Stir onions into mixture and let it sit for 5 minutes. Heat about 1 inch of oil to 350° F in a skillet over high heat.
- When the oil is very hot, drop a small mound of onion rings into the oil. Press down slightly with spatula. Fry on one side until crisp and brown, turn over and fry second side. Remove bhajis as they cook. Keep warm in 200F oven. Pile on platter with mango chutney.

Onion Brie Appetizers

Makes 18 servings

Ingredients:
- 2 medium onions - thinly sliced
- 3 tablespoons butter or margarine
- 2 tablespoons brown sugar
- 1/2 teaspoon cider vinegar
- 1 sheet frozen puff pastry - thawed
- 4 ounces Brie, rind removed - softened
- 1/2 teaspoon caraway seeds
- 1 egg
- 2 teaspoons water

Directions:
- In a large skillet, cook the onions, butter, brown sugar and vinegar over medium low heat until onions are golden brown, stirring frequently. Remove with a slotted spoon; cool to room temperature.
- On a lightly floured surface, roll puff pastry into an 11 x 8" rectangle. Spread Brie over pastry. Cover with the onions and sprinkle with caraway seeds. Roll up one long side to the middle of the dough. Roll up the other side so the two rolls meet in the center.
- Using a serrated knife, cut into 1/2" slices. Place on parchment paper lined baking sheets. Flatten to 1/4" thickness. Refrigerate for 30 minutes.
- In a small bowl, beat egg and water; brush over slices. Bake at 375 for 12 minutes or until puffed and golden brown. Serve warm.

Onion Jam Appetizer On Toast Points

Makes 8 servings

Ingredients:
- 3 tablespoons butter
- 4 large onions - thinly sliced
- 1/2 teaspoon lite salt (to taste)
- 1/4 teaspoon pepper (to taste)
- 1 baguette - sliced and toasted

Directions:
- In a large skillet, melt the butter and add the onions, salt, and pepper. Cook over medium heat, stirring often, for 20 minutes.
- Turn up the heat and continue cooking, stirring occasionally, for 20 minutes more or until the onions have melted.
- Spoon the onion mixture onto the toast points and serve at once.

Roasted Tomato, Onion & Goat Cheese Frittatini

Makes 24 servings

Ingredients:
- 4 roma tomatoes
- Lite salt and pepper - to taste
- 4 tablespoons extra virgin olive oil
- Vegetable shortening - as needed
- 1/2 red onion - finely diced
- 5 eggs
- 2 fluid ounces 2% milk
- 3 tablespoons parmesan cheese -- grated
- 1 tablespoon fresh basil leaves -- chopped
- 2 ounces goat cheese - crumbled

Directions:
- Quarter the tomatoes and squeeze out the excess juice. Toss the tomatoes with salt, pepper and a small amount of the olive oil. Spread them on a sheet pan and roast in a 350F oven for 20 minutes.
- Allow the tomatoes to cool, then chop coarsely.
- Brush muffin cups well with the vegetable shortening.
- Heat the remaining olive oil in a small sauté pan. Add the onion and cook until translucent but not brown. Remove from the heat and cool to room temperature

(continued)
- In a medium bowl, beat the eggs. Beat in the milk, then add the parmesan, onion, chopped

basil, goat cheese and tomatoes. Season with salt and pepper and stir well.
- Fill the prepared muffin tins one-third full with the mixture. Bake at 350F until the frittatini are golden and feel firm to the touch. Cool slightly, carefully unmold and serve warm.
- Serve one frittatini per person garnished with fresh basil leaves and accompanied by approximately 1/4 cup of dressed mixed greens salad.

Gingered Mango Salsa

Makes 10-12 servings

Ingredients:
- 2 cups chopped peeled mango
- 1/2 cup chopped Vidalia onion
- 1/2 cup minced fresh cilantro
- 1/2 cup lime juice
- 1/4 cup minced fresh mint
- 2 tablespoons minced fresh ginger root
- 1 teaspoon olive oil
- 1/2 teaspoon salt

Directions:
- In a bowl, combine all ingredients. Let stand for 30 minutes before serving.

Greek Style Avocado Dip

Makes 12 servings

Ingredients:
- 2 1/2 avocado - peeled, pitted and diced
- 2 1/2 cloves garlic, minced
- 1/4 cup and 2 teaspoons lime juice
- 2 1/2 roma (plum) tomato, seeded and diced
- 1/2 cup and 1 tablespoon, 2 teaspoons crumbled feta cheese

Directions:
- Mash together the avocado, garlic, and lime juice in a bowl until nearly smooth. Fold in the diced tomato and feta cheese.

Fruit Guacamole

Makes 10 servings

Ingredients:
- 1 avocado - peeled, pitted, and diced

- 1 1/2 teaspoons minced red onion
- 1 teaspoon minced seeded serrano chile
- 12 red grapes, halved
- 1/2 cup fresh diced peaches
- Salt to taste
- 2 tablespoons pomegranate seeds (optional)

Directions:
- Gently mash the avocado with the onion and serrano pepper in a bowl. Mix in the grapes and peaches. Season with salt and, if desired, garnish with pomegranate seeds to serve.

Chocolate Covered Strawberries

Makes 24 servings

Ingredients:
- 16 ounces milk chocolate chips
- 2 tablespoons shortening
- 1 pound fresh strawberries with leaves

Directions:
- Insert toothpicks into the tops of the strawberries.
- In a double boiler, melt the chocolate and shortening, stirring occasionally until smooth. Holding them by the toothpicks, dip the strawberries into the chocolate mixture.
- Turn the strawberries upside down and insert the toothpick into styrofoam for the chocolate to cool.

Jalapeno Hummus

Makes 15-20 servings

Ingredients:
- 1 3/4 cups and 2 tablespoons garbanzo beans
- 1/2 cup and 2 tablespoons canned or fresh jalapeno pepper slices, juice reserved
- 1/3 cup and 1 teaspoon tahini
- 5 1/2 cloves garlic, minced
- 3 tablespoons and 2 1/4 teaspoons lemon juice
- 1 teaspoon ground cumin
- 1 teaspoon curry powder (optional)
- Crushed red pepper to taste

Directions:
- In a blender or food processor, mix the garbanzo beans, jalapeno peppers and reserved juice, tahini, garlic, and lemon juice. Season with cumin, curry powder, and crushed red pepper. Blend until smooth.

Mexican Layered Dip

Makes 10-15 servings

Ingredients:
- 1 (16 ounce) can refried beans
- 1 (1.25 ounce) package taco seasoning mix
- 1 large tomato, seeded and chopped
- 1 cup guacamole
- 1 cup sour cream, room temperature
- 1 cup shredded sharp Cheddar cheese
- 1/3 cup chopped green onions
- 1/4 cup chopped black olives

Directions:
- Spread refried beans in the bottom of a (1-quart) shallow edged serving dish (you can use a transparent dish if you'd like). Sprinkle the seasoning packet over the beans. Layer the diced tomatoes over the beans, the sour cream over the tomatoes, and the guacamole over the sour cream. Sprinkle the entire layered dip with cheddar cheese, followed by green onion and finishing it off with a layer of black olives. Cover and refrigerate until ready to serve.

Coffee Flavored Fruit Dip

Makes 32 servings

Ingredients:
- 1 (8 ounce) package cream cheese, softened
- 1 (8 ounce) container sour cream
- 1/2 cup brown sugar
- 1/3 cup coffee-flavored liqueur
- 1 (8 ounce) container frozen whipped topping, thawed

Directions:
- Place cream cheese, sour cream, brown sugar and coffee-flavored liqueur in a medium bowl. Blend together with an electric mixer until smooth. Fold in thawed frozen whipped topping. Chill in the refrigerator until serving.

Fruit Dip

Makes 24 servings

Ingredients:
- 8 ounces cream cheese, softened
- 1/2 cup marshmallow creme

- 2 cups frozen whipped topping, thawed
- 1/4 cup unsweetened pineapple juice

Directions:
- Blend together the cream cheese, marshmallow cream and thawed topping. Add enough pineapple juice to make it dipping consistency. Chill for 1 hour.

Grilled Fruit Sates

Makes 24 servings

Ingredients:
- 1 cup and 2 tablespoons white sugar
- 4 1/2 cups balsamic vinegar
- 1/4 cup freshly ground black peppercorns
- 12 large fresh peaches with peel, halved and pitted
- Fresh Cantaloupe, cubed
- Fresh Pineapple, cubed
- 15 ounces blue cheese, crumbled

Directions:
- In a saucepan over medium heat, stir together the white sugar, balsamic vinegar, and pepper. Simmer until liquid has reduced by one half. It should become slightly thicker. Remove from heat, and set aside.
- Preheat grill for medium-high heat.
- Lace cantaloupe, pineapple cubes and peaches on skewers. Lightly oil the grill grate. Place pineapple and peaches on the prepared grill, cut side down. Cook for about 5 minutes, or until the flesh is caramelized. Turn over. Brush the top sides with the balsamic glaze, and cook for another 2 to 3 minutes.
- Transfer the fruit to individual serving dishes, and drizzle with remaining glaze. Sprinkle with crumbled blue cheese.

Apple Gouda Quesadillas

Makes 35-40 servings

Ingredients:
- 40 (8 inch) flour tortillas
- 1/2 cup and 2 tablespoons olive oil
- 1/2 cup and 2 tablespoons Dijon mustard
- 10 green onions, chopped
- 10 red apples, cored and thinly sliced
- 10 cups shredded Gouda cheese

Directions:
- Preheat a grill for high heat.
- Brush oil onto one side of a tortilla, and place on a plate oil side down. Spread about 1/2 tablespoon of mustard on the top side, and top with green onion, apple slices and about 1/2 cup of shredded cheese. Place a second tortilla on top, and brush the top with olive oil. Repeat with remaining ingredients, stacking the quesadillas on the plate.
- Brush the grilling surface with oil, and place the quesadillas carefully on the grill. Grill for about 3 minutes, or until the bottom is crisp. Flip, and grill on the other side until crisp. Remove from the grill to serving plates and cut into quarters. Serve warm.

Double Tomato Bruschetta

Makes 12 servings

Ingredients:
- 6 roma (plum) tomatoes - chopped
- 1/2 cup sun-dried tomatoes - packed in oil
- 3 cloves minced garlic
- 1/4 cup olive oil
- 2 tablespoons balsamic vinegar
- 1/4 cup fresh basil, stems removed
- 1/4 teaspoon salt
- 1/4 tsp ground black pepper
- 1 French baguette
- 2 cups shredded mozzarella cheese

Directions:
- Preheat the oven on broiler setting.
- In a large bowl, combine the roma tomatoes, sun-dried tomatoes, garlic, olive oil, vinegar, basil, salt, and pepper. Allow the mixture to sit for 10 minutes.
- Cut the baguette into 3/4-inch slices. On a baking sheet, arrange the baguette slices in a single layer. Broil for 1 to 2 minutes, until slightly brown.
- Divide the tomato mixture evenly over the baguette slices. Top the slices with mozzarella cheese.
- Broil for 5 minutes, or until the cheese is melted.

Chicken and Sun-Dried Tomato Bruschetta

Makes 15 servings

Ingredients:
- 4 skinless, boneless chicken breast halves
- 2-1/2 cups Italian salad dressing, divided
- 8 cups fresh spinach, torn

- 2/3 cup crumbled feta cheese
- 16 sun-dried tomatoes, packed without oil, chopped
- 2 (1 pound) loaves focaccia bread, cut into 1/2-inch thick slices
- 1/2 cup olive oil

Directions:
- Place the chicken and 1 cup salad dressing in a bowl. Cover, and marinate at least 3 hours in the refrigerator.
- Preheat the grill for high heat.
- Lightly oil the grill grate. Discard dressing used for marinating, and grill chicken 7 minutes per side, or until juices run clear. Cool and shred.
- In a large bowl, mix the cooked chicken, spinach, feta cheese, sun-dried tomatoes, and remaining dressing.
- Brush the focaccia bread with olive oil, and cook 1 minute per side on the prepared grill, or until lightly toasted. Place portions of the chicken mixture on the toasted focaccia to serve.

Spinach & Cheddar Whole Wheat Quesadillas

Makes 15-20 servings

Ingredients:
- 10 (10 inch) whole wheat tortillas
- 15 cups fresh spinach leaves
- 3-1/3 cups shredded Cheddar cheese
- 5 green onion, chopped
- 2-1/2 teaspoons garlic powder
- 2-1/2 teaspoons chili powder

Directions:
- Heat a large non-stick skillet over medium-high heat. Place 1 tortilla onto the skillet. Sprinkle about half the Cheddar cheese evenly over the tortilla. Top with the spinach, green onions, garlic powder, and chili powder. Cover with the remaining Cheddar cheese. Place the second tortilla on top.
- Cook until the bottom tortilla starts to develop a bit of color and starts to crisp, about 3 minutes. To flip and cook the other side, slide the quesadilla off the non-stick pan onto a dinner plate, cover with another dinner plate and flip. The crispy tortilla side should now be on top. Slide the quesadilla back onto the pan and cook until the bottom tortilla starts turning crisp, about 3 minutes more. Slide onto a cutting board, and cut into 8 wedges to serve.

Alaskan Spicy Spinach Dip

Makes 12 servings

Ingredients:
- 2 pounds pepperjack cheese

- 2 cups half-and-half cream
- 1 large tomato, diced
- 1 onion, diced
- 1/2 cup diced red bell pepper
- 3 cups spinach, rinsed and chopped

Directions:
- Over a double boiler slowly melt the pepperjack cheese. When the cheese is melted whisk in half and half until smooth and creamy. Stir in tomato, onion, red bell pepper and chopped spinach. Transfer to a serving bowl. Serve warm with tortilla chips or bread.

So Cheesy Beer & Spinach Dip

Makes 36 servings

Ingredients:
- 2/3 cup beer
- 3 cups shredded Monterey Jack cheese
- 2 tablespoons all-purpose flour
- 1/2 cup frozen chopped spinach, thawed and drained
- 1 tablespoon chopped fresh cilantro
- Salt and pepper (to taste)

Directions:
- In a medium saucepan over medium heat, bring beer to a boil. Lower heat. Slowly stir in Monterey Jack cheese and flour. Cook and stir until cheese is melted but not bubbly.
- Mix spinach, cilantro, salt and pepper into the beer mixture. Serve warm.

Orange and Rosemary Baked Olives

Makes 12-15 servings

Ingredients:
- 3 1/2 cups whole mixed olives, drained
- 1/4 cup dry white wine
- 2 tablespoons fresh orange juice
- 2 tablespoons olive oil
- 2 cloves garlic, minced
- 2 sprigs fresh rosemary
- 2 tablespoons fresh parsley, chopped
- 1 1/2 tablespoons chopped fresh oregano
- 4 teaspoons grated orange zest
- 1/4 teaspoon crushed red pepper flakes

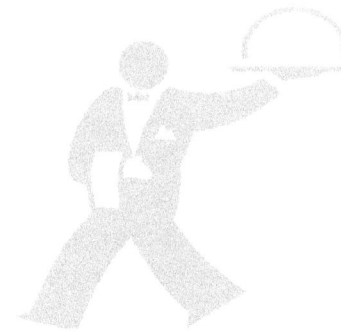

Directions:
- Preheat oven to 375° F (190° C). Stir the olives together with the wine, orange juice, olive oil, and garlic in a 9x13 inch baking dish. Nestle the sprigs of rosemary in the olives.
- Bake in the preheated oven for 15 minutes, stirring halfway through the baking. Remove and discard the rosemary sprigs, then stir in the parsley, oregano, orange zest, and red pepper flakes. Serve warm, or cool, or use them to top a salad.

Bacon Olive Wraps

Makes 15-20 servings

Note: You'll need toothpicks to secure the wraps.

Ingredients:
- 10 slices white bread, crusts trimmed
- 1 (16 ounce) jar processed cheese sauce
- 1 (5 ounce) jar pitted green olives, chopped
- 1 pound sliced bacon, cut in half

Directions:
- Preheat the broiler.
- Cut bread into thirds. Spread each third with processed cheese sauce. Sprinkle with olives. Roll thirds jelly-roll fashion. Wrap each with half a strip of bacon, securing with toothpicks. Arrange wrapped bread rolls in a single layer on a large baking sheet.
- Broil, checking frequently, until bacon is evenly browned and has reached desired crispness, about 5 minutes.

Olive Pecan Spread

Makes 12-15 servings

Ingredients:
- 8 ounces cream cheese, softened
- 1/2 cup mayonnaise
- 1 (5 ounce) jar sliced green olives, drained
- 1 cup coarsely chopped pecans

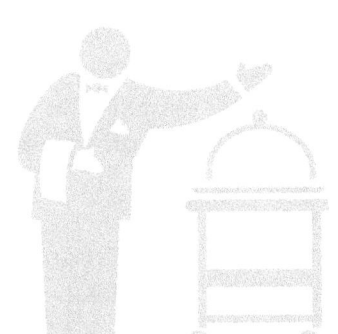

Directions:
- Mix together the cream cheese, mayonnaise, olives and pecans in a bowl. Refrigerate at least 1 hour before serving.

Caribbean Fruity Salsa

Makes 16-20 servings

Ingredients:
- 2 cups diced fresh mango
- 1 cup diced fresh pineapple
- 1 cup diced papaya
- 2 fresh jalapeno pepper, seeded and minced
- 1 medium red onion, finely diced
- 1/4 cup lime juice
- 2 tablespoons olive oil
- 2 teaspoons salt, or to taste
- 2 tablespoons chopped fresh mint

Directions:
- Toss together the mango, pineapple, papaya, jalapeno pepper, and red onion in a medium bowl. Pour in the lime juice and olive oil. Season to taste with salt, and stir to combine. Sprinkle with chopped mint leaves before serving. Note: Serve as a fruit salad or is great for breakfast with yogurt and granola

Mississippi Caliente Caviar

Makes 15 servings

Ingredients:
- 3 (15 ounce) cans black-eyed peas
- 1 cup diced green chili peppers
- 3/4 cup diced onion
- 3/4 cup diced jalapeno chile pepper
- 1/4 cup diced pimento peppers, drained
- 1 1/2 teaspoons minced garlic
- 1 (16 ounce) bottle Italian-style salad dressing

Directions:
- In a mixing bowl, combine the black-eyed peas, green chili pepper, onion, jalapeno pepper, pimento, garlic and Italian-style dressing. Chill the mixture overnight.

Strawberry Bread

Makes 2 loaves

Ingredients:
- 2 10 oz. packages frozen strawberries, thawed

- 3 cups flour
- 1 teaspoon baking powder
- 1/2 teaspoon salt
- 1 1/2 teaspoons cinnamon
- 2 cups sugar
- 3 eggs, beaten
- 1 cup veg. oil
- 1 cup chopped pecans

Directions:
- Preheat oven to 350° F. Drain strawberries, reserving 1/2 cup juice. Mix together the flour, baking soda, salt, cinnamon and sugar. Make a hole in the center of mixture and pour in strawberries, oil, eggs, and pecans. Mix by hand until thoroughly combined. Pour into 2 greased and floured loaf pans. Bake 40-60 minutes.

Spread:
- 1/2 c. strawberry juice
- 1 8 oz. package cream cheese
- Blend together the strawberry juice and cream cheese til spreading consistency. Serve as a spread for the cooled and sliced bread.

Pineapple Cheese Spread

Makes 5 cups

Ingredients:
- 2 8 ounce cream cheese
- 1 8 1/2 ounce can crushed pineapple, drained
- 1 cup chopped pecans
- 1/2 cup chopped green bell pepper
- 2 tablespoons chopped green onion
- 1 teaspoon Lawry's Seasoned Salt

Directions:
- Soften cream cheese and mix with pineapple, nuts, green pepper and onions. Blend in salt and mix well. Pack into a crock and refrigerate to set or roll into a ball covered with crushed pecans. Serve with crackers.

Stuffed Cherry Tomatoes

Makes 12-16 servings

Ingredients:
- 2 pkgs. (one 8 ounces, and one 3 ounces) cream cheese, softened

- 2 tablespoons mayonnaise
- 1 pkg (.4 ounce) ranch salad dressing mix
- 3 dozen cherry tomatoes

Directions:
- In a mixing bowl, blend cream cheese, mayonnaise and salad dressing mix until smooth. slice a thin slice off tops of tomatoes and carefully remove insides; invert on paper towel to drain. Fill with cream cheese mixture.

Strawberry-Cheese Ball

Ingredients:
- 1 cup mayonnaise
- 1 1/2 cup sharp cheddar cheese
- 1/2 cup chopped pecans
- 2 green onions, chopped

Directions:
- Mix in ball and refrigerate overnight. Pour 5 oz. strawberry preserves over ball just before serving. Serve with a butter cracker such as Ritz.

Spirited Apricot Brie

Makes 6 servings

Ingredients:
- 1/2 cup apricot jam
- 1 tablespoon grated orange peel
- 1 tablespoon brandy or orange juice
- 1 tablespoon lemon juice
- 1/8 teaspoon ground cinnamon
- 1 piece brie cheese (about 1/2 lbs.)
- Thin baguette slices or water crackers

Directions:
- Mix jam, orange peel, brandy, lemon juice, and cinnamon in a shallow microwave-safe serving dish just large enough to also hold the brie.
- Set brie in apricot sauce. Return to microwave oven and cook, uncovered, until the cheese is hot and slightly melted, about 1 minute; check at 20-second intervals.
- Scoop cheese and apricot sauce onto the baguette slices.

COLDFINGERFOODS
COLDFINGERFOODS
COLDFINGERFOODS
COLDFINGERFOODS
COLDFINGERFOODS
COLDFINGERFOODS
COLDFINGERFOODS

COLD FINGER FOODS

COLDFINGERFOODS
COLDFINGERFOODS
COLDFINGERFOODS
COLDFINGERFOODS
COLDFINGERFOODS
COLDFINGERFOODS
COLDFINGERFOODS
COLDFINGERFOODS
COLDFINGERFOODS

Wonton Wrapper Appetizers

Makes 60 servings

Ingredients:
- 1 (16 ounce) package wonton wrappers
- 1 pound sausage
- 1 cup shredded Monterey Jack cheese
- 1 cup shredded Cheddar cheese
- 1/2 cup chopped black olives, drained
- 1 cup Ranch-style salad dressing

Directions:
- Preheat oven to 350° F (175° C). Spray a miniature muffin pan with cooking spray.
- Insert wonton wrappers into the muffin pan so as to form small cups. Bake 5 minutes in the preheated oven. Allow the baked wrappers to cool. Remove from the pan.
- In a medium bowl, mix the sausage, Monterey Jack, Cheddar, black olives and Ranch-style dressing. Fill the baked wonton wrapper cups with the mixture.
- Bake the filled wonton wrappers 10 to 15 minutes, until the sausage mixture is bubbly and slightly brown. Watch closely so the wonton wrappers do not burn.

Cajun Deviled Eggs

Makes 24 servings

Ingredients:
- 12 eggs
- 1/4 cup mayonnaise
- 2 teaspoons prepared Dijon-style mustard
- 1/2 teaspoon salt
- 1/2 teaspoon ground black pepper
- 1/2 teaspoon ground cayenne pepper

Directions:
- Place eggs in a medium saucepan and cover with cold water. Bring water to a boil and immediately remove from heat. Cover and let eggs stand in hot water for 10 to 12 minutes. Remove from hot water, cool and peel.
- Slice eggs in half lengthwise. Remove yolks and place in a medium bowl. Set aside egg whites. Mashing with a fork, mix mayonnaise, Dijon-style mustard, salt and black pepper with the egg yolks.
- Fill the hollowed egg white halves with the yolk mixture. Sprinkle with cayenne pepper, adjusting the amount to taste. Cover and chill in the refrigerator until serving. Note: Put egg mixture in a Ziplock bag, press all of the air out of the bag and seal. Cut the tip of the bag off and use as a pastry bag to fill the egg whites.

Guacamole Deviled Eggs

Makes 12 servings

Ingredients:
- 6 hard boiled eggs - halved lengthwise and yolk removed
- 2 tablespoon Dukes mayonnaise
- 1 tablespoon fresh lime juice
- 2 avocado- peeled, pitted and mashed
- 1 tablespoon cilantro - finely chopped
- 1 tablespoon sweet onion - finely chopped
- 1 tablespoon tomato- finely diced
- Kosher salt (to taste)
- Black pepper (to taste)

Directions:
- Cut eggs in half lengthwise. Remove yolks and set whites aside. Mash yolks with fork. Stir in remaining ingredients until well blended. Refill whites, using about 1 tablespoon yolk mixture for each egg half. Chill to blend flavors.
- Quick-and-easy method: Cut eggs in half lengthwise. Remove yolks and place in 1-quart plastic food storage bag. Set whites aside. Add remaining ingredients. Press out air. Seal bag. Press and roll bag until yolk mixture is well blended. Push yolk mixture toward bottom corner of bag. Snip off about 1/2 inch of bag corner.
- Squeezing bag gently from the top, fill reserved whites with yolk mixture. Chill to blend flavors.

Salsa Deviled Eggs

Ingredients:
- 6 hard boiled eggs
- 2 tablespoon Dukes Mayonnaise
- 2 tablespoon tomato - finely diced
- 1 tablespoon chile peppers - finely chopped
- 2 tablespoon sweet onion - finely diced
- 1/2 teaspoon apple cider vinegar
- Kosher salt (to taste)
- Black pepper (to taste)

Directions:
- Cut eggs in half lengthwise. Remove yolks and set whites aside. Mash yolks with fork. Stir in remaining ingredients until well blended. Refill whites, using about 1 tablespoon yolk mixture for each egg half. Chill to blend flavors.
- Quick-and-easy method: Cut eggs in half lengthwise. Remove yolks and place in 1-quart plastic food storage bag. Set whites aside. Add remaining ingredients. Press out air. Seal bag. Press and roll bag until yolk mixture is well blended. Push yolk mixture toward bottom corner of bag.

Snip off about 1/2 inch of bag corner.
- Squeezing bag gently from the top, fill reserved whites with yolk mixture. Chill to blend flavors.

Pesto Deviled Eggs

Makes 12 servings

Ingredients:
- 6 hard-cooked eggs
- 3 tablespoons grated Parmesan cheese
- 2 tablespoons plain low-fat yogurt
- 1 teaspoon basil leaves, crushed
- 1/2 teaspoon garlic powder

Directions:
- Cut eggs in half lengthwise. Remove yolks and set whites aside. Mash yolks with fork. Stir in remaining ingredients until well blended. Refill whites, using about 1 tablespoon yolk mixture for each egg half. Chill to blend flavors.
- Quick-and-easy method: Cut eggs in half lengthwise. Remove yolks and place in 1-quart plastic food storage bag. Set whites aside. Add remaining ingredients. Press out air. Seal bag. Press and roll bag until yolk mixture is well blended. Push yolk mixture toward bottom corner of bag. Snip off about 1/2 inch of bag corner.
- Squeezing bag gently from the top, fill reserved whites with yolk mixture. Chill to blend flavors.

Wrap-and-Roll Basil Pinwheels

Makes about 24 pinwheels

Ingredients:
- 3 (7 or 8 inch) flour tortillas
- 1 (5.2 ounce) carton Boursin Cheese or one 5 ounce. container semi soft cheese with garlic and herbs
- 12 large fresh basil leaves
- 1/2 of a 7 ounce jar roasted red sweet peppers, cut into 1/4 inch wide strips
- 4 ounces thinly sliced cooked roast beef, ham, or turkey
- 1 tablespoon Dukes mayonnaise
- Fresh basil leaves

Directions:
- Spread each flour tortilla with 1/3 of the Boursin cheese or semisoft cheese with garlic and herbs. Add a layer of the large fresh basil leaves to cover cheese. Divide roasted red sweet pepper strips between the tortillas; arrange roasted red pepper strips over the basil leaves 1 to 2 inches apart. Top with meat slices. Spread 1 teaspoon mayonnaise over the meat on each tortilla. Roll up the tortillas tightly, jell-roll style, enclosing the filling. Wrap each roll in plastic wrap.

Chill the tortilla rolls in the refrigerator 2 to 4 hours to blend flavors.

• To serve, remove the rolls from the refrigerator. Remove the plastic wrap from the tortilla rolls; cut each of the rolls into 1-inch slices (make diagonal slices, if desired). Garnish with the fresh basil leaves, if you wish. Skewer each of the cut tortilla rolls on frilly picks or on short decorative skewers, if desired.

Spinach Roll-Ups

Ingredients:
- 2 boxes frozen spinach, defrost and squeeze out the liquid
- 1 cup mayonnaise
- 1 cup sour cream
- 1 cup Baco Bits
- 1/2 pkg Buttermilk Ranch Dressing
- Flour tortillas

Directions:
• Mix together first 5 ingredients. Spread on flour tortillas and roll up. Wrap in wax paper. Refrigerate overnight. Slice and serve.

Potato Hummus

Ingredients:
- 1 pound potatoes (3 medium), peeled and cut into 1-inch cubes
- 4 large cloves garlic
- 1/2 to 3/4 cup roasted sesame tahini (available in Middle Eastern stores)
- 1/3 cup fresh lemon juice
- 1/4 cup olive oil
- 2/3 cup water
- 1 teaspoon ground cumin
- 1/2 teaspoon cayenne pepper
- 2 teaspoons kosher salt
- Red, green and yellow bell pepper strips
- Pita bread, cut into wedges

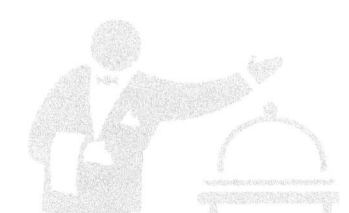

Directions:
• In a heavy saucepan with a tight-fitting lid, cook the potatoes and garlic in 2 inches of salted boiling water until tender, approximately 15 minutes.

• Drain thoroughly and pass through a ricer or food mill into a bowl. Add the tahini, lemon juice and oil and blend thoroughly. Gradually stir in the water until the mixture is the proper consistency for dipping. Add the cumin and cayenne, then season with salt.

• Serve with pepper strips and wedges of pita bread.

Baba Ganouj

Ingredients:
- 1 medium size eggplant
- 1 clove garlic
- Juice of 1 small lemon
- 1 tablespoon tahini (sesame paste)
- 1 tablespoon olive oil
- Salt and freshly-ground pepper

Directions:
- Roast eggplant in a 450° F oven for 30 to 40 minutes, turning once, or until flesh is very tender and a sharp knife pierces without resistance.
- When cool enough to handle, remove peel. In a food processor, mince garlic. Add eggplant flesh, lemon juice, tahini and olive oil. Process to blend (may be smooth or a little chunky). Add salt and pepper to taste.
- Serve with fresh or toasted pita bread.

Skordalia (Greek)

Ingredients:
- 4 thick slices bread, soaked in water
- 1 1/2 cups mashed cooked potatoes
- 3 cloves garlic
- 1/2 cup walnuts
- 3/4 cup olive oil
- 1/3 cup fresh lemon juice
- 1/2 teaspoon salt

Directions:
- Squeeze bread to remove excess water. Place bread, potatoes, garlic and walnuts in food processor. Whirl until smooth and creamy. With machine running, add oil in slow, steady stream through feed tube until thoroughly incorporated. Blend in lemon juice and salt.
- Serve in bowl with vegetables or triangles of pita bread for dipping.

Chocolate Cheese Cake Dip

Makes 3 3/4 cups of dip, or 6 servings

Ingredients:
- 1/2 cup raisins
- 1 tablespoon brandy
- 2 cups cream cheese, softened
- 1/2 cup whipping cream

- 1 teaspoon vanilla extract
- 1/4 cup dark brown sugar
- 1 teaspoon ground cinnamon
- 1/2 cup miniature chocolate chips
- Ground cinnamon

Directions:
- Mix the raisins and brandy, making sure all the raisins are coated, and let soak for 15 minutes. In another bowl, beat the cream cheese and whipping cream until well blended and smooth. Add vanilla extract, mixing well. Blend in the brown sugar and cinnamon. Mix in the "soused" raisins and chocolate chips, blending well. Garnish with a light dusting of cinnamon. Serve at room temperature.

Suggested dippers:
- Graham crackers, melon, strawberries, raspberries, peaches, pears, dried fruit, pound cake cubes

Jalapeno Jelly Cheese Loaf

- Put 1 (8 ounce) block of cream cheese on a nice serving plate. Spread jalapeno jelly over the top of the cream cheese, letting it run down the sides and onto the plate. Serve with assorted crackers.

Buttery Blue Cheese Spread with Walnuts

Makes 5 cups, or 24 servings

Ingredients:
- 24 ounces cream cheese, softened
- 1/2 cup butter, softened
- 4 ounces crumbled blue cheese
- 1 cup diced walnuts, toasted
- 1/2 cup chopped fresh chives
- 1/4 cup cream sherry
- 1 (16 ounce) round bread loaf
- Garnishes: toasted diced walnuts, chopped fresh chives, rosemary sprigs

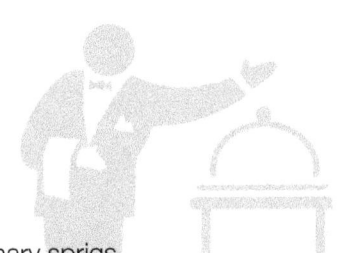

Directions:
- Stir together first 5 ingredients and, if desired, sherry in a large bowl; cover and chill mixture 8 hours.
- Let stand at room temperature to soften; or freeze spread up to 1 month, and thaw in the refrigerator for 8 hours.
- Hollow out bread loaf, leaving a 1-inch-thick shell; reserve inside of loaf for other uses. Spoon softened cheese spread into shell. Garnish, if desired. Serve with sliced apples and pears or

HOT FINGER FOODS

Baked Cream Cheese Wontons

Makes 16 servings

Ingredients:
- 32 wonton wrappers (Nasoya All Natural Wonton Wraps)
- 6 tbsps cream cheese
- Pam cooking spray
- 8 tablespoons duck sauce

Directions:
- Preheat oven to 400° F.
- Place about 1/2 tsp cream cheese in the center of a wonton wrapper. Wet your finger with water and moisten the edges of the wrapper. Fold wonton in half to make a triangle, sealing the cream in the wonton well (the water acts like glue). Moisten one corner of the wonton with more water. Bring the bottom edges of the won ton together, overlapping slightly to form a wonton appetizer shape. If you like, you can skip this step and just make triangles. Repeat for the rest of the wontons.
- Place won tons on a nonstick cookie sheet sprayed with Pam. Spray wontons with a bit of Pam. It seems weird, but it helps the wontons brown in the oven. Bake won tons at 400° F for 7-12 minutes or until golden brown and crispy.
- Serve wontons with duck sauce for dipping.

Spinach Brownies

Makes 24 servings

Ingredients:
- 1 (10 ounce) package spinach, rinsed and chopped
- 1 cup all-purpose flour
- 1 teaspoon kosher salt
- 1 teaspoon baking powder
- 2 eggs
- 1 cup fat free milk
- 1/2 cup butter, melted
- 1 sweet onion, chopped
- 1 (8 ounce) package shredded mozzarella cheese

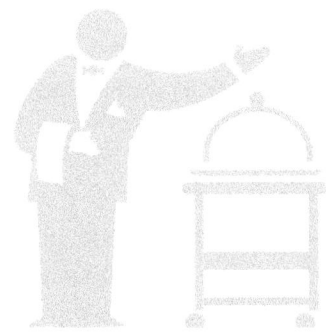

Directions:
- Preheat oven to 375° F (190° C). Lightly grease a 9x13 inch baking dish.
- Place spinach in a medium saucepan with enough water to cover. Bring to a boil. Lower heat to simmer and cook until spinach is limp, about 3 minutes. Remove from heat and set aside.
- In a large bowl, mix flour, salt, and baking powder. Stir in eggs, milk and butter. Mix in spinach, onion and mozzarella.

• Transfer the mixture to the prepared baking dish. Bake in the preheated oven 30-35 minutes, or until a toothpick inserted in the center comes out clean. Cool before serving.

Pigs in a Blanket

Makes 16 servings

Ingredients:
- 2 8 ounce tubes of crescent roll dough
- 3 ounce cheddar cheese (shredded)
- 16 cocktail franks
- 1/4 cup heavy cream
- Your favorite mustard

Directions:
- Preheat your oven to 400° F.
- Next, unroll the tubes of crescent roll dough and separate each triangle. You should have 8 triangles per tube. Then, slice off 1/2 inch of the dough on the LONG end and discard.
- Sprinkle the dough with the shredded cheese (about 1 teaspoon for each triangle). Place a cocktail frank at the base of each triangle and roll up away from you, enclosing the frank in the dough. This makes the Pigs in Blankets. Trim each off the excess dough at both ends.
- Place each piggy 2 inches apart on a cookie sheet lined with parchment paper. Position them so that the tip is on the top.
- Then, lightly brush the top of each with the heavy cream and place the cookie sheet in the oven. Bake until golden brown and a little puffed up - about 15 minutes.

Super Sausage Balls

Makes 48 pieces

Ingredients:
- 2 packages of refrigerated crescent rolls
- 1 package cocktail franks or sausage (fully cooked)

Directions:
- Preheat oven to 375° F.
- Next, separate the dough into 6-8 triangles. Then, cut each triangle into thirds (lengthwise.) You and your child can easily place the little franks on the short end of each triangle and then it roll up to the opposite point. Finally, place each rolled frank on an ungreased cookie sheet.
- All you need to do now is bake the franks for 12 to 15 minutes or until the crescent rolls have turned a golden brown. Serve on your favorite serving platter.

Hot Artichoke Dip

Ingredients:
- Tortilla chip strips (for dipping)
- Crudités (vegetables for dipping: carrots, celery, cauliflower, broccoli, etc.)
- 14 ounces marinated artichoke hearts
- 1 (4 ounce) can mild green chilies
- 1 (2 ounce) jar chopped pimentos
- 1 jar La Victoria salsa (or equivalent)
- Cilantro
- 1/2 cup grated Jack or cheddar cheese
- 2 tablespoons mayonnaise (optional)
- 2 tablespoons sour cream (optional)

Directions:
- Drain and chop artichoke hearts, mild green chilies and pimentos. Combine above ingredients in a large bowl. Add salsa to taste, add mayonnaise and sour cream. Place in a small casserole dish or quiche dish.
- Top with grated cheese and microwave covered 4 to 6 minutes until bubbly. Garnish with sour cream, cilantro and olives.
- Serve with tortilla strips and crudités or fill cooked artichokes with hot dip.

Cheese Ball Pastry

Makes 24 servings

Ingredients:
- 1/2 cup of soft sharp cheddar cheese (jar cheese works best)
- 3 tablespoons butter
- 3/4 cup of flour
- 1/2 teaspoon kosher salt
- 1/2 teaspoon paprika
- 1/2 teaspoon curry

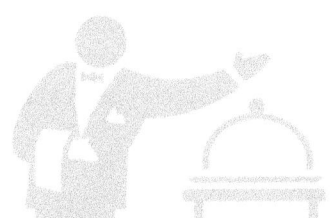

Directions:
- Preheat oven to 400° F. Cream together cheese and butter. Sift together remaining ingredients. Add sifted flour ingredients to cheese mixture, blend well.
- Pinch off pieces of dough, then roll to form approximately 3/4-inch diameter cheese balls. Chill for 2 hours.
- Place cheese balls on an un-greased cookie sheet. Bake about 10 minutes. Serve hot.

Jalapeno Sausage Poppers

Makes 20 pieces

Ingredients:
- 1 (10 ounce) pkg. Butterball turkey sausage links or patties (or equivalent fully-cooked turkey sausage)
- 8 ounces pepper jack cheese (shredded)
- 1 (4 ounce) container jalapeno peppers (chopped and drained)
- 1 (10 count) can flaky ready-to-bake biscuits

Directions:
- Thaw sausage if frozen. Use a food processor to chop sausage to a crumble mixture.
- In a large bowl, combine crumbled sausage, cheese and drained jalapeno peppers (add jalapeno peppers according to your taste).
- Separate each biscuit into 2 halves, making 20 separate pieces. Shape each piece into a square approximately 3" x 3". Put sausage mixture in each square, then pinch together like dumplings.
- Place on cookie sheet and bake according to biscuit directions. Serve warm or cold.
- Serve with dip consisting of 8 ounces of sour cream mixed with 1 package of taco seasoning.

Tomato and Onion Tart

Ingredients:
- 7 sheets phyllo dough, thawed
- 1/2 stick of butter, melted
- 5 6 ounce bag/container fresh-grated parmesan cheese
- 1 medium sweet onion, thinly sliced
- 2 cups shredded provolone cheese
- 5-6 plum (Roma) tomatoes, cut into 1/8-in.-thick slices
- 8-10 fresh basil leaves, snipped fine
- Kosher salt and freshly ground black pepper

Directions:
- Preheat oven to 375° F.
- Line a large baking sheet with parchment paper and spray paper with nonstick cooking spray. Lay 1 sheet phyllo dough on paper and brush lightly with a little melted butter. Sprinkle top of buttered phyllo with 1-2 tablespoons fresh parmesan, using enough to cover all areas but not overload it. Repeat layering 6 more times (phyllo, butter, and parmesan), pressing each sheet so it sticks to the sheet below.
- Lay onion slices on top of the parmesan cheese, (you can use as many as you want) and top with the shredded provolone. Arrange tomato slices in a single layer on top of the provolone, edge to edge. Sprinkle surface with the fresh basil, and salt and pepper to taste.
- Bake for 30 minutes. Allow to cool 10 minutes, then cut and serve.

Cheese Triangles

Makes 32 servings

Ingredients:
- 2 cups all-purpose flour
- 2 teaspoons baking powder
- 3/4 teaspoons ground red pepper (optional)
- 1/2 teaspoon salt
- 3 tablespoons shortening
- 1/2 cup finely shredded sharp cheddar cheese (2 ounces)
- 3/4 cup milk
- 1 tablespoon milk
- 1/2 cup finely shredded sharp cheddar cheese (2 ounces)

Directions:
- Preheat oven to 400° F. Lightly grease baking sheets; set aside. In a large bowl stir together flour, baking powder, red pepper (if using), and salt. Using a pastry blender, cut in shortening until the size of coarse crumbs. Stir in 1/2 cup finely shredded cheese. Add the 3/4 cup milk, stirring just until dry ingredients are moistened. Form into a ball.
- On a lightly floured surface, roll dough to a 10-inch square, 1/4 inch thick. Brush with the 1 tablespoon milk and sprinkle with 1/2 cup finely shredded cheese; press lightly. Cut into sixteen 2-1/2-inch squares. Cut each square in half diagonally to make 32 triangles. Place on the prepared baking sheets.
- Bake about 12 to 15 minutes or until golden brown. Serve warm.

Herb and Cheese Mini Quiche

Makes 40 servings

Ingredients:
- 1 cup butter, softened
- 2 3-ounce packages cream cheese, softened
- 2 cups all-purpose flour
- 1/4 cup shredded Asiago cheese (1 ounce)
- 2 eggs, beaten
- 1/2 cup half-and-half
- 1/4 cup finely shredded Gouda or Havarti cheese
- 2 tablespoons pine nuts, toasted and coarsely chopped
- 1 tablespoon snipped fresh tarragon or 2 teaspoons dried tarragon, crushed
- 1 tablespoon snipped fresh chives
- 1/8 teaspoon cracked black pepper
- Roasted red pepper, finely chopped

- Snipped fresh chives

Directions:
- Preheat oven to 325° F. For pastry, in a large bowl, beat the butter and cream cheese with an electric mixer on medium to high speed for 30 seconds. Beat in the flour and Asiago cheese until a soft dough forms. Press 1 rounded teaspoon of the pastry evenly into the bottom and up the side of each of 48 ungreased 1-3/4-inch muffin cups.
- For filling, in a medium bowl, stir together eggs; half-and-half; Gouda or Havarti cheese; pine nuts; tarragon; the 1 tablespoon chives; and the black pepper.
- Spoon about 1 heaping teaspoon of the filling into each pastry-lined muffin cup. Bake in the preheated oven for 25 to 30 minutes or until a knife inserted in centers comes out clean. Cool slightly in muffin cups. Carefully remove from muffin cups; place on a wire rack or serving platter. Top with chopped roasted red pepper and additional snipped chives. Serve warm.

Gougeres

Makes 60 pieces

Ingredients:
- 1 1/2 cups water
- 1/2 cup butter, cut into pieces
- 1/4 teaspoon kosher salt
- 1 1/2 cups all-purpose flour
- 5 eggs
- 1 1/2 cups shredded Gruyere cheese (6 ounces)
- 4 teaspoons Dijon-style mustard
- 1/8 teaspoon ground white pepper
- 1/4 teaspoon cayenne pepper

Directions:
- Lightly grease two baking sheets; set aside. In a medium saucepan, combine the water, butter, and salt. Bring to boiling. Add flour all at once, stirring vigorously. Cook and stir until mixture forms a ball. Remove from heat. Transfer to a large mixing bowl. Cool for 10 minutes. Add eggs, one at a time, beating with an electric mixer on medium speed for 1 minute after each addition. Stir in Gruyere cheese, mustard, white pepper, and the 1/8 teaspoon cayenne pepper.
- Preheat oven to 400° F. Using a pastry bag fitted with a 1/2-inch star tip, pipe batter in 1-inch mounds about 1 1/2 inches apart onto the prepared baking sheets. (Or use 2 teaspoons batter for each puff.)
- Bake for 20 to 25 minutes or until puffed and golden brown. Serve warm. If desired, sprinkle with additional cayenne pepper.

FOWLTREATS
FOWLTREATS
FOWLTREATS
FOWLTREATS
FOWLTREATS
FOWLTREATS
FOWLTREATS

FOWL TREATS

FOWLTREATS
FOWLTREATS
FOWLTREATS
FOWLTREATS
FOWLTREATS
FOWLTREATS
FOWLTREATS
FOWLTREATS

Buffalo Chicken Dip

Ingredients:

- 4 boneless skinless chicken breast halves, boiled, drained and shredded with 2 forks
- 1 (12 ounce) bottle Frank's Hot Sauce
- 16 ounces cream cheese
- 1 (16 ounce) bottle Ranch dressing
- 1/2 cup minced celery
- 8 ounces shredded Monterey jack or sharp Cheddar cheese

Directions:
- Preheat oven to 350° F.
- In a 13 x 9 x 2-inch baking pan, combine the shredded chicken meat with entire bottle of Frank's hot sauce, spreading to form an even layer.
- In a large saucepan over medium heat, combine the cream cheese with entire bottle of Ranch dressing, stirring until smooth and hot. Pour evenly over the chicken mixture. Sprinkle celery over top.
- Bake uncovered for 20 minutes, then sprinkle cheese over top and bake uncovered for another 15 or 20 minutes until just hot and bubbly. Let stand 10 minutes before serving with celery sticks or any sturdy dipping chip.

Chicken Satay Appetizers

Ingredients:
- 1 pound skinless boneless chicken breasts, cut into 24 cubes*
- 4 tablespoons soy sauce, divided
- 1/4 cup peanut butter
- 2 tablespoons honey
- 1 tablespoon Oriental sesame oil
- 1 (12 ounce) bottle chili sauce
- 3 tablespoons chopped fresh parsley
- 1 medium red, green or yellow bell pepper, cut into 24 (1-inch) squares

Directions:
- Marinate chicken in 2 tablespoons soy sauce for 15 minutes.
- Meanwhile, for sauce, thoroughly combine the remaining soy sauce, peanut butter, honey and oil; stir in chili sauce and parsley and set aside.
- Thread a piece of chicken and bell pepper square onto small bamboo skewers that have been soaked in water. Broil 4 inches from heat source for 6 minutes, turning once. Serve with sauce.

*1 pound boneless pork loin may be substituted. Slice 1/2 inch thick; cut slices into 1/4-inch strips.

Chili Chicken Strips

Ingredients:
- 1/4 cup sour cream
- 3/4 cup fresh salsa
- 1 pound boneless, skinless chicken breasts
- 1 egg
- 4 cups Fritos
- 1 teaspoon chili powder
- 3 cups canola oil

Directions:
- In a small bowl, combine sour cream and salsa. Refrigerate, covered, until ready to serve.
- Cut chicken into approximately 24 strips. Beat egg in a shallow bowl. In another shallow bowl, crush Fritos and stir in chili powder. Dip chicken strips in egg, then coat with seasoned crushed Fritos. Refrigerate until ready to use (up to 2 days).
- In a deep, heavy skillet, heat oil to 375° F. Fry chicken strips a few at a time until golden brown. Drain on paper towels. Note: If you don't have a deep-fat thermometer, drop a 1-inch cube of bread in the oil. If it turns golden brown in 1 minute, the oil is hot enough.
- Serve hot with creamy salsa.

Pecan Crusted Chicken Fingers

Ingredients:
- 3 skinless, boneless chicken breast halves,
- 2 teaspoons Cajun spice
- 1/2 teaspoon kosher salt
- 1/2 teaspoon Cajun seasoning
- 4 tablespoons pecan meal or 2 tablespoons pecan halves, finely ground
- 1 egg white
- 2 teaspoons canola oil
- Apricot Sauce
- 1 cup canned apricot nectar
- 2 tablespoons spicy mustard
- 1 tablespoons cider vinegar
- 1 teaspoon cornstarch

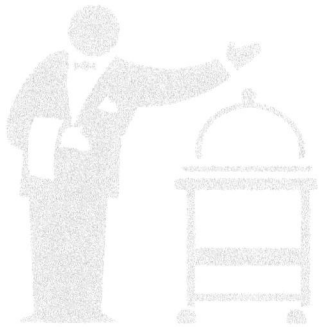

Directions:
- Slice chicken into 1/2 inch wide strips. Set aside.
- Beat the egg white lightly in a wide, shallow dish.
- In another dish, mix together the spices and the pecan meal. Dip each chicken strip in the egg white, then roll lightly in the pecan-spice mixture. Set on wax paper. If not cooking immediately, refrigerate, uncovered.
- Heat canola oil in skillet over medium-high heat. Cook without crowding, turning occasion-

ally, until chicken is opaque, firm to the touch, and pecan meal is golden brown. Drain on paper towels. Serve with apricot sauce.

Apricot Sauce:
- Combine apricot nectar and spicy mustard in small saucepan. Stir to blend and bring to boil over medium heat.
- In small dish combine the vinegar and cornstarch to make paste. Add to boiling nectar, stir until slightly thickened; serve warm.

Red Hot Chicken Bits

Ingredients:
- 3 pound boned chicken breasts
- 1/8 teaspoon garlic salt
- 2 tablespoons red pepper
- 1/2 teaspoon black pepper
- 1 cup flour
- Canola oil

Directions:
- Cut chicken breasts lengthwise into 1-inch pieces. Sprinkle garlic salt freely over chicken, turning pieces so each is coated. Continue with red, then black pepper. Set aside for 1 hour to let chicken absorb flavor. Dust chicken with flour, then deep fry in oil at 375° F for 3 minutes. Drain on paper towels.
- Serve warm or cold.

Chili Chicken Strips

Ingredients:
- 1/4 cup sour cream
- 3/4 cup fresh salsa
- 1 pound boneless, skinless chicken breasts
- 1 egg
- 4 cup Fritos
- 1 teaspoon chili powder
- 3 cups canola oil

Directions:
- In a small bowl, combine sour cream and salsa. Refrigerate, covered, until ready to serve.
- Cut chicken into approximately 24 strips. Beat egg in a shallow bowl. In another shallow bowl, crush Fritos and stir in chili powder. Dip chicken strips in egg, then coat with seasoned crushed Fritos. Refrigerate until ready to use (up to 2 days).
- In a deep, heavy skillet, heat oil to 375° F. Fry chicken strips a few at a time until golden brown. Drain on paper towels. Note: If you don't have a deep-fat thermometer, drop a 1 inch

cube of bread in the oil. If it turns golden brown in 1 minute, the oil is hot enough.
- Serve hot with creamy salsa.

Honey Mustard Drummettes

Ingredients
- 40 chicken wing drumettes
- 2/3 cup honey
- 6 tablespoons Dijon mustard
- 6 tablespoons soy sauce

Directions
- In ungreased 12x8-inch (2-quart) glass baking dish, arrange chicken drumettes in single layer.
- In 1-cup microwave-safe measuring cup, combine honey, mustard and soy sauce; mix well. Microwave on HIGH for 30 seconds. Stir until well blended. Drizzle honey mixture over chicken, brushing as necessary to coat chicken. If desired, cover and refrigerate up to 2 hours.
- Heat oven to 375° F. Uncover dish; turn chicken drumettes. Bake 50 to 60 minutes or until chicken is tender, glazed and no longer pink next to bone, turning chicken once halfway through baking time.
- Just before serving, brush with honey mixture from dish.

Mandarin Chicken Bites

Makes 15 servings

Ingredients:
- 1 cup of flour (all-purpose)
- 1 teaspoon of kosher salt
- 1 teaspoon of fresh cracked pepper
- 1 pound of chicken breasts (boneless, skinless)
- 2 tablespoons of butter (or margarine)
- 1 11-ounce can of mandarin oranges (drained)
- 2/3 cup of orange marmalade
- 1/2 teaspoon of dried tarragon

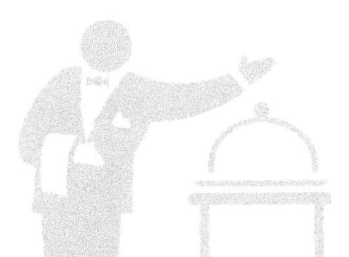

Directions:
- The first thing to do is cut the chicken into bite-size pieces. Then, combine the salt and pepper and flour in a large plastic bag (resealable). Adding a few pieces of chicken at a time, shake to coat. Remove the chicken pieces and brown them in a skillet in melted butter. When the juices run clear, you've cooked the chicken long enough.
- Next, in a small saucepan, mix the oranges, marmalade and tarragon and then bring the mixture to a boil.
- Simply, pour the mixture over the chicken and stir everything gently to coat it all.

Transfer the coated chicken to a pretty platter and serve warm with some toothpicks.

BEEFTREATS
BEEFTREATS
BEEFTREATS
BEEFTREATS
BEEFTREATS
BEEFTREATS
BEEFTREATS

BEEF TREATS

BEEFTREATS
BEEFTREATS
BEEFTREATS
BEEFTREATS
BEEFTREATS
BEEFTREATS
BEEFTREATS

Jamaican Meat Patties

Makes 12 medium, 6 large, or 24 appetizer servings

Ingredients:
Basic Pie Pastry
- 1 1/2 teaspoon curry powder, lite salt and pepper to taste to pastry recipe
- 2 cups flour
- 1/2 cup white vegetable shortening or margarine
- 5 tablespoons ice water
- Curry powder as above
- Lite salt and pepper

Filling
- 1 pound ground beef (turkey or chicken)
- 1 small onion fine chopped
- 1/2 red bell pepper chopped
- 1 large clove garlic minced
- 1 teaspoon thyme
- 2 teaspoons curry powder
- Few drops of hot pepper sauce to taste
- 2 teaspoons Worcestershire sauce
- 1/4 cup beef broth
- 1/4 cup flour

Directions:
- Make standard pastry and chill wrapped about 4 hour or overnight. Make filling by sauteing in olive oil, onions, peppers, and garlic until softened. Add ground meat and cook and stir and break up meat until meat is browned and cooked. Add remaining ingredients and cook and stir until mixture is fully cooked and thickened. Remove from heat, adjust seasonings and cool. Remove pastry from refrigerator and let soften at room temperature about 15 minutes. Roll pastry out on lightly floured surface to 1/4 inch thick. Cut out circles with a 4 inch circular cutter or cut size as desired. Place some filling in center of circle and fold over edges to seal and prick edges with tinges of a fork. Bake 400° F until golden, (about 15 mins. for small pieces, 20 mins for medium pieces and 25 to 30 mins for larger pieces).

Orange Glazed Cocktail Sausages

Makes 25 servings

Ingredients:
- 1 package Lit'l Smokies (50 links)
- 1 cup brown sugar
- 1 tablespoon flour
- 2 tablespoons mustard

- 1 tablespoon vinegar
- 1/4 cup orange juice concentrate (undiluted)

Directions:
- Combine ingredients and heat until warm in microwave.

Mexican Beef Egg Rolls

Makes 20 servings

Ingredients
- 1/4 cup vegetable oil
- 2 pounds ground beef
- 2 large onion, chopped
- 10 cloves garlic, minced
- 2 red bell pepper, chopped
- 2 (1 ounce) packages taco seasoning
- 2 (8 ounce) jars taco sauce
- 8 (16 ounce) packages egg roll wrappers
- 2 (1 pound) loaves Velveeta, cut into 1/4 inch thick slices
- 4 egg whites, lightly beaten
- 16 cups canola oil

Directions:
- Place the vegetable oil and ground beef into a large skillet; cook over medium-high heat until the meat is evenly browned and no longer pink. Reduce the heat to medium. Mix in the onion, garlic, and bell pepper; cook until the vegetables are softened, about 5 minutes. Stir in the taco seasoning and taco sauce. Continue to cook and stir the mixture until the sauce begins to bubble, about 5 minutes more.
- Working on a clean, flat surface, place 1 egg roll wrapper with a corner facing you. Place 1 tablespoon of the meat mixture in the center of the wrapper and top with a slice of cheese. Fold the corner closest to you over the meat mixture and roll the wrapper over the mixture 1-1/2 times. Fold in the two opposite side corners and continue rolling the wrapper so it covers these corners, tucking them in. Dip two fingers in the egg whites and brush the remaining corner, pressing it to seal. Repeat these steps with a second egg roll wrapper. Let the egg roll rest briefly so the egg white dries and holds the last corner in place.
- If the egg rolls will not be served right away, preheat oven to 325° F (165° C). Line a heat-proof dish with paper towels.
- Pour the canola oil into a large wok set over medium-high heat. When the oil begins to shimmer, carefully slip two to three egg rolls into the wok. Cook until the wrappers turn golden brown and bubble slightly, 30 seconds to 1 minute. Use a slotted spoon or strainer to remove from the wok. Place the egg rolls in the prepared dish and put the dish in the heated oven, making sure to remove it after 15 minute or lower the temperature. Continue cooking the remaining egg rolls.

Java Style Beef Sate

Makes 16 servings

Ingredients
- 2 heads garlic, peeled
- 10 shallots, chopped
- 2 (1 inch) pieces galangal, thinly sliced
- 16 red chile peppers, seeded and chopped
- 2 cups roasted macadamia nuts
- 2 teaspoons belacan shrimp paste
- 1/2 cup vegetable oil
- 4 pounds boneless beef sirloin steak, cut into 1/2 inch cubes
- 4 cups water
- 1/4 cup palm sugar
- 2 beef bouillon cube
- 2 tablespoons salt
- 1/4 cup and 2 tablespoons kecap manis
- 12 kaffir lime leaves, finely chopped
- 64 wooden skewers, soaked in water for 15 minutes

Directions:
- In a mortar with a pestle, mash together the garlic, shallots, galangal, chile peppers, and macadamia nuts into a fine paste. Add the shrimp paste and oil, continue mashing until incorporated. Place the paste into a large skillet over medium-high heat, cook and stir until fragrant, about 3 minutes.
- Stir the beef into the sauce and cook for 5 minutes, stirring constantly. Pour in the water, palm sugar, bouillon cube, and salt. Simmer until the water has evaporated, about 10 minutes, stirring frequently. Stir in the kecap manis and lime leaves, then spread the beef out on a baking sheet or large dish, and allow to cool until cool enough to handle.
- Preheat an outdoor grill for medium-high heat, and lightly oil the grate. Remove the beef cubes from the tray, and thread onto skewers, reserve any leftover sauce for basting.
- Cook on preheated grill for a few minutes until slightly browned; baste occasionally with the leftover sauce.

Beef Spring Rolls with Carrots and Cilantro

Makes 16 servings

Ingredients:
- 3 3/4 pounds beef top sirloin or top round steak, cut 3/4 to 1 inch thick or flank steak
- 3/4 cup and 3 tablespoons stir-fry sauce and marinade
- 30 rice paper wrappers (8 to 9 inch diameter)
- 3 3/4 cups shredded carrots

- 3 3/4 cups lightly packed fresh cilantro
- 2/3 cup and 2 teaspoons stir-fry sauce and marinade
- Additional prepared stir-fry sauce and marinade

Directions:
- Cut beef steak lengthwise in half, then crosswise into 1/8 to 1/4-inch thick strips. Combine 1/4 cup stir-fry sauce and beef in medium bowl. Cover and marinate in refrigerator 30 minutes to 2 hours.
- Heat large nonstick skillet over medium-high heat until hot. Add 1/2 of beef; stir-fry 1 to 3 minutes or until outside surface of beef is no longer pink. (Do not overcook.) Remove from skillet. Repeat with remaining beef.
- Fill large bowl with warm water. Dip 1 rice paper wrapper into water for a few seconds or just until moistened. Rice paper will still be firm but will continue to soften during assembly. Place on work surface.
- Spoon 1/4 cup beef, 2 tablespoons carrots and 2 tablespoons cilantro evenly in a row across center of wrapper, leaving 1 inch border on right and left sides; drizzle with about 1 teaspoon reserved stir-fry sauce. Fold right and left sides of wrapper over filling. Fold bottom edge up over filling and roll up tightly. Repeat with remaining wrappers and filling ingredients. Cut each spring roll diagonally in half. Serve with additional stir-fry sauce, if desired.

Cocktail Meatballs

Makes 15 servings

Ingredients:
- 1 1/2 pounds lean ground beef
- 1 1/2 egg
- 3 tablespoons water
- 3/4 cup bread crumbs
- 1/4 cup and 1 teaspoon minced onion
- 1 1/2 (8 ounce) cans jellied cranberry sauce
- 1 cup and 2 tablespoons chili sauce
- 1 tablespoon plus 1-1/2 teaspoons brown sugar
- 2-1/4 teaspoons lemon juice

Directions:
- Preheat oven to 350° F (175° C).
- In a large bowl, mix together the ground beef, egg, water, bread crumbs, and minced onion. Roll into small meatballs.
- Bake in preheated oven for 20 to 25 minutes, turning once.
- In a slow cooker or large saucepan over low heat, blend the cranberry sauce, chili sauce, brown sugar, and lemon juice. Add meatballs, and simmer for 1 hour before serving.

Sweet and Sour Meatballs

Makes 15 servings

Ingredients
- 3 3/4 pounds lean ground beef
- 3 3/4 eggs
- 1 3/4 cups and 2 tablespoons dry bread crumbs
- 3/4 cup and 3 tablespoons finely chopped onion
- 1 teaspoon ground ginger
- 1-3/4 teaspoons seasoning salt
- 1 teaspoon ground black pepper
- 1 tablespoon and 3/4 teaspoon Worcestershire sauce
- 1 tablespoon and 3/4 teaspoon granulated sugar
- 2 (20 ounce) cans pineapple chunks, drained with juice reserved
- 1/2 cup and 2 tablespoons water
- 1/3 cup and 1 teaspoon distilled white vinegar
- 1 tablespoon and 2-1/2 teaspoons soy sauce
- 3/4 cup and 3 tablespoons packed brown sugar
- 1/3 cup and 1 teaspoon cornstarch
- 1 teaspoon ground ginger
- 1 teaspoon seasoning salt
- 2 large carrot, diced
- 2 large green bell pepper, cut into 1/2 inch pieces

Directions:
- Preheat oven to 400° F (200° C). Lightly grease a large, shallow baking sheet.
- In a large bowl, thoroughly mix the ground beef, eggs, bread crumbs and onion. Sprinkle with ginger, seasoning salt, pepper, Worcestershire sauce and sugar. Shape into one inch balls.
- Place meatballs in a single layer on prepared baking sheet. Bake in preheated oven for 10 to 15 minutes; set aside.
- To make the sauce, mix enough water with the reserved pineapple juice to make 1 cup. In a large pot over medium heat, combine the juice mixture, 1/3 cup water, vinegar, soy sauce, and brown sugar. Stir in cornstarch, ginger and seasoning salt, until smooth. Cover and cook until thickened.
- Stir pineapple chunks, carrot, green pepper and meatballs into the sauce. Gently stir to coat the meatballs with the sauce. Simmer, uncovered, for about 20 minutes, or until meatballs are thoroughly cooked.

Veal, Beef, and Pork Meatballs

Makes 15 servings

Ingredients:
- 2 pounds ground beef
- 15 ounces ground veal
- 15 ounces ground pork
- 3 3/4 cloves garlic, minced
- 3 3/4 eggs
- 1 3/4 cups and 2 tablespoons freshly grated Romano cheese
- 2 tablespoons and 2 1/2 teaspoons chopped Italian flat leaf parsley
- salt and ground black pepper to taste
- 3 3/4 cups stale Italian bread, crumbled
- 2 3/4 cups and 1 tablespoon lukewarm water
- 1 3/4 cups and 2 tablespoons olive oil

Directions:
- Combine beef, veal, and pork in a large bowl. Add garlic, eggs, cheese, parsley, salt and pepper.
- Blend bread crumbs into meat mixture. Slowly add the water 1/2 cup at a time. The mixture should be very moist but still hold its shape if rolled into meatballs. (I usually use about 1 1/4 cups of water). Shape into meatballs.
- Heat olive oil in a large skillet. Fry meatballs in batches. When the meatball is very brown and slightly crisp remove from the heat and drain on a paper towel. If your mixture is too wet, cover the meatballs while they are cooking so that they hold their shape better.

Grilled Sirloin Kabobs

Makes 16 servings

Ingredients:
- 1/2 cup soy sauce
- 1/4 cup and 2 tablespoons light brown sugar
- 1/4 cup and 2 tablespoons distilled white vinegar
- 1 teaspoon garlic powder
- 1 teaspoon seasoned salt
- 1 teaspoon garlic pepper seasoning
- 1 cup lemon-lime flavored carbonated beverage
- 4 pounds beef sirloin steak, cut into 1 1/2 inch cubes
- 4 green bell peppers, cut into 2 inch pieces
- skewers
- 1 pound fresh mushrooms, stems removed
- 4 cups cherry tomatoes

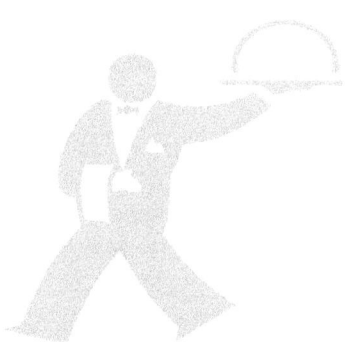

- 2 fresh pineapple - peeled, cored and cubed

Directions:
- In a medium bowl, mix soy sauce, light brown sugar, distilled white vinegar, garlic powder, seasoned salt, garlic pepper seasoning, and lemon-lime flavored carbonated beverage. Reserve about 1/2 cup of this marinade for basting. Place steak in a large resealable plastic bag. Cover with the remaining marinade, and seal. Refrigerate for 8 hours, or overnight.
- Bring a saucepan of water to a boil. Add green peppers, and cook for 1 minute, just to blanch. Drain, and set aside.
- Preheat grill for high heat. Thread steak, green peppers, mushrooms, tomatoes, and pineapple onto skewers in an alternating fashion. Discard marinade and the bag.
- Lightly oil the grill grate. Cook kabobs on the prepared grill for 10 minutes, or to desired doneness. Baste frequently with reserved marinade during the last 5 minutes of cooking.

Corned Beef Bagel Dip

Makes 16 servings

Ingredients:
- 3/4 cup Miracle Whip
- 3/4 cup sour cream
- 2 (2.5 ounce) packages thinly sliced deli corned beef, chopped
- 1/4 cup chopped onion
- 1 tablespoon minced fresh parsley
- 1/2 teaspoon seasoned salt
- 2 teaspoons prepared horseradish (optional)
- 3 bagels, cut into bite-size pieces

Directions:
- In a bowl, combine mayonnaise and sour cream. Stir in the corned beef, onion, parsley, seasoned salt and horseradish. Serve with bagel pieces.

Corned Beef Party Puffs

Makes 12 servings

Ingredients:
- 2 1/2 cups finely chopped deli corned beef
- 2 tablespoons chopped onion
- 2 tablespoons Dijon mustard
- 1 tablespoon mayonnaise
- 1/4 teaspoon prepared horseradish
- 1 cup beer
- 1/2 cup butter

- 1 cup flour
- 1/4 teaspoon salt
- 4 eggs

Directions:
- Mix together the corned beef, onion, mustard, mayonnaise, and horseradish. Cover and refrigerate.
- Preheat an oven to 450° F (230° C).
- In a large pot, bring beer and butter to a rolling boil. Stir in flour and salt until the mixture forms a ball. Transfer the dough to a large mixing bowl. Using a wooden spoon or stand mixer, beat in the eggs one at a time, mixing well after each. Drop by teaspoonfuls onto a lightly greased baking sheet.
- Bake for 10 minutes in the preheated oven. Reduce temperature to 350° F (175° C) and bake an additional 10 minutes until golden brown. Centers should be dry.
- When the shells are cool, split the puffs and fill with the corned beef mixture. Refrigerate until ready to serve.

Beefy Cheese Ball

Ingredients:
- 1 jar sliced dried beef, rinsed and finely chopped
- 8 ounces cream cheese, softened
- 1/4 cup dairy sour cream
- 1/4 cup grated Parmesan cheese
- 2 teaspoons prepared horseradish

Directions:
- Combine 1/4 cup of the dried beef, cream cheese, sour cream, Parmesan cheese and horseradish; blend thoroughly. Refrigerate mixture for 15 minutes.
- Form into a ball and roll in remaining dried beef. Chill thoroughly.
- Serve with crackers.

SEAFOOD FARE

Herbed Shrimp On Grits Cakes

Ingredients:
- 3 cups instant grits
- 1/4 cup butter
- 1 cup shredded Gruyere cheese
- 3 pounds fresh shrimp, tails on, deveined (16-18 count)
- 1/3 cup extra virgin olive oil
- 1 tablespoon chopped fresh dill
- 1 tablespoon chopped fresh parsley
- 1 tablespoon chopped fresh chives
- 1 teaspoon sea salt
- 1 teaspoon fresh cracked pepper
- 1 lemon – grate peel

Directions:
- Cook grits per package instructions and then stir in butter and cheese.
- Pour mixture into a jelly roll pan and cover with plastic wrap. Refrigerate for 3-4 hours until set.
- Using a 2 inch fluted round cutter, cut rounds from the grits and set aside.
- In a medium bowl, combine the shrimp, olive oil, dill, parsley, chives, salt , pepper, then toss to coat well with PAM and add shrimp.
- Cook until pink and remove from heat.
- Top each grits cake with one shrimp and garnish with fresh grated lemon peel.
- Serve immediately.

Crab Cake Bites

Makes 48 servings

Ingredients:
- 2 celery stalks
- 2 whole eggs
- 1/4 cup mayonnaise
- 1/4 cup dry white wine
- 1 teaspoon freshly ground black pepper
- 1 teaspoon kosher salt
- 1/2 teaspoon cayenne pepper
- 1 tablespoon Maryland crab seasoning
- 1 1/2 pounds cooked crabmeat, flaked
- 2 cups unsalted panko bread crumbs
- 1 large sweet onion- grated
- 1/4 cup fresh parsley, minced
- 2 egg whites

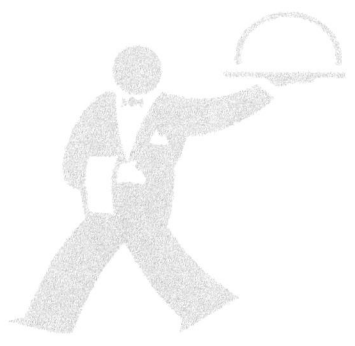

- 3 tablespoons extra virgin olive oil
- 3 tablespoons unsalted butter
- Maryland Crab Dipping Sauce – recipe below

Directions:
- Remove strings from celery and cut into small diced pieces. In a large bowl, mix whole eggs, mayonnaise, wine, black pepper, salt, cayenne pepper, and Maryland Crab Seasoning.
- Add crabmeat, bread crumbs, onion, celery and parsley. Whisk egg whites until foamy, then fold into crab mixture.
- Heat oil and butter in a large skillet and drop tablespoonfuls of crab cakes into hot pan. Cook 3 minutes or until browned. Turn and cook 3 minutes on the other side. Drain on paper towels.

Maryland Crab Dipping Sauce

Makes 3 cups

Ingredients:
- 1 cup mayonnaise
- 1/2 cup prepared mild mustard
- 3/4 ketchup
- 1/2 cup drained sweet pickle relish
- 1/4 cup bottled horseradish
- 1 tablespoon Maryland Crab Seasoning
- 1/2 teaspoon Texas Pete hot sauce

Directions:
- Mix all ingredients with a wire whisk and chill until ready to serve.

Smoked Salmon Triangles

Makes 50 servings

Ingredients:
- 25 slices packaged thin-sliced cocktail bread
- 12 ounces cream cheese
- 3 tablespoons sour cream
- 2 tablespoons red horseradish
- 2 lemons
- 8 ounce smoked salmon
- 50 capers, drained
- Olives
- Parsley and thin lemon slices for garnish

Directions:
- Trim crusts from bread and cut in half diagonally. Mix cream cheese, sour cream, and undrained horseradish. Spread thinly on bread.
- Trim ends from lemons and slice paper thin with a sharp knife. Cut slices into wedges. Cut salmon slices into triangles and place on cheese mixture. Top each with a piece of lemon and a caper.
- Accompany with assorted olives and garnish with parsley and lemon slices.

Mini Blinis with Caviar

Makes 40 servings

Ingredients:
- 1 envelope active dry yeast
- 1 teaspoon sugar
- 1/2 cup very warm water
- 1 cup King Arthur plain flour
- 2 cups buckwheat flour
- 1 cup buttermilk
- 1 cup water
- 2 eggs, separated
- 1 teaspoon baking soda
- 1/2 cup molasses
- 5 tablespoons butter, melted and cooled
- Additional butter for skillet
- 1 pint sour cream
- 8 ounces caviar

Directions:
- Proof yeast with sugar in warm water for 10 minutes.
- Mix flours and add to a large bowl with yeast mixture, buttermilk, and water. Stir till blended and cover and let stand for one hour or refrigerate for 6-8 hours until ready to cook.
- Beat egg whites until stiff and set aside. Add the baking soda to molasses and set aside. Beat egg yolk and melted butter into batter and then incorporate molasses and whites. Drop by tablespoonfuls onto lightly buttered skillet. Cook until edges bubble. Turn blini and cook about 30 seconds longer. Remove to warm platter and top each with a teaspoon of sour cream and then 1/2 teaspoon of caviar.

Ceviche

Ingredients:
- 1 pound bay scallops
- 8 limes, juiced
- 2 tomatoes, diced

- 5 green onions, minced
- 2 stalks celery, sliced
- 1/2 green bell pepper, minced
- 1/2 cup chopped fresh parsley
- freshly ground black pepper
- 1 1/2 tablespoons olive oil
- 1/8 cup chopped fresh cilantro

Directions:
- Rinse scallops and place in a medium sized bowl. Pour lime juice over the scallops. The scallops should be completely immersed in the lime juice. Chill the lime juice and scallops all day or overnight until scallops are opaque (you cannot see through them).
- Empty 1/2 of the lime juice from the bowl. Add tomatoes, green onions, celery, green bell pepper, parsley, black pepper, olive oil, and cilantro to the scallop mixture. Stir gently. Serve this dish in fancy glasses with a slice of lime hanging over the rim for effect. Note: You may substitute many types of seafood for scallops, for example: halibut, red snapper, flounder, or swordfish.

Catfish Mini Cakes

Makes 40 servings

Ingredients:
- 5 pounds catfish fillets
- 5 medium onion, chopped
- 1 tablespoon and 2 teaspoons prepared yellow mustard
- 1/4 cup and 1 tablespoon creamy salad dressing (Miracle Whip)
- 2 1/2 teaspoons Old Bay Seasoning, or to taste
- 12 1/2 cups coarsely crushed Ritz Crackers
- 5 eggs
- 5 cups canola oil (for frying)

Directions:
- Place catfish in a saucepan with enough water to cover. Bring to a boil, and cook until fish flakes easily with a fork. Drain off water, and mash up the fish. Stir in the onion, mustard, salad dressing, Old Bay™, cracker crumbs and egg. Mix until evenly blended.
- Heat oil in a large heavy skillet over medium-high heat. Form the fish mixture into patties, and fry in the hot oil. Drain on paper towels, and serve hot.

Vietnamese Salad Rolls

Ingredients:
- 1 (8 ounce) package rice vermicelli
- 8 ounces cooked, peeled shrimp, cut in half lengthwise
- 8 rice wrappers (6.5 inch diameter)

- 1 carrot, julienned
- 1 cup shredded lettuce
- 1/4 cup chopped fresh basil
- 1/2 cup Peking sauce
- Water as needed

Directions:
- Bring a medium saucepan of water to boil. Remove from heat. Place rice vermicelli in boiling water, remove from heat, and let soak 3 to 5 minutes, until soft. Drain, and rinse with cold water.
- Fill a large bowl with hot water. Dip one rice wrapper in the hot water for 1 second to soften. Lay wrapper flat, and place desired amounts of noodles, shrimp, carrot, lettuce and basil in the center. Roll the edges of the wrapper slightly inward. Beginning at the bottom edge of wrapper, tightly wrap the ingredients. Repeat with remaining ingredients.
- In a small bowl, mix the Peking sauce with water until desired consistency has been attained. Heat the mixture for a few seconds in the microwave.
- Serve the spring rolls with the warm dipping sauce.

Lobster Fritters

Ingredients:
- 1 cup chopped Lobster
- 2 Eggs
- 1/2 cup milk
- 1 1/4 cups Flour
- 2 teaspoons baking powder
- Salt and pepper (to taste)
- Canola Oil
- Lemon wedges

Directions:
- Heat deep frying oil to 350-375° F. While fat is heating, beat eggs until light. Add milk and flour sifted with baking powder, salt and pepper, then fold in chopped lobster. Drop by small spoonfuls into oil and fry until golden brown. Drain on rack in warm oven. Serve lobster fritters with lemon wedges and your favorite dipping sauce.

Leftover Salmon Patties

Ingredients:
- Leftover baked salmon
- Leftover mashed potatoes
- 1 to 2 eggs
- Flour
- Butter
- Salt and pepper (to taste)

Directions:
- Flake leftover salmon into a large bowl. Add potatoes, salt, and pepper. You can also add other seasonings at this time to your liking. Beat the egg(s) lightly in a separate bowl, then stir into the fish-potato mixture. The mix should not be too moist. Form into balls, roll in flour, then flatten into patties. In a skillet, saute salmon patties in melted butter over medium to hot heat. Turn cakes to brown on both sides.

Muffin Pan Crab Cakes

Ingredients:
- 1 pound crabmeat
- 2 cups fresh breadcrumbs
- 1/2 red bell pepper, minced
- 3 scallions, sliced
- 1/4 cup Dukes mayonnaise
- 2 large eggs
- 1 large egg white
- 10 dashes Texas Pete hot sauce
- 1/2 teaspoon celery salt
- 1/4 teaspoon freshly ground pepper
- 1 teaspoon Old Bay
- 6 lemon wedges for garnish

To make fresh breadcrumbs: Trim crusts from firm sandwich bread. Tear bread into pieces and process in a food processor until a coarse crumb forms. One slice of bread makes about 1/3 cup crumbs.

Directions:
- Preheat oven to 450° F.
- Generously coat a 12-cup nonstick muffin pan with cooking spray.
- Mix crab, breadcrumbs, bell pepper, scallions, mayonnaise, eggs, egg white, hot sauce, celery salt, Old Bay and pepper in a large bowl until well combined. Divide mixture evenly among muffin cups. Bake until crispy and cooked through, 20 to 25 minutes. Serve with lemon wedges.

Shrimp and Crab Cakes

Ingredients:
- 8 ounces finely chopped cooked shrimp
- 8 ounces lump crabmeat, cleaned and picked over to remove any bits of shell
- 2 teaspoons Dijon-style mustard
- 1/4 cup Dukes mayonnaise
- 2 tablespoons minced fresh parsley
- 2 teaspoons worcestershire sauce
- 1/2 teaspoon Tabasco sauce
- 2 teaspoons bottled white horseradish

- Kosher salt
- Cayenne pepper (to taste)
- 1/4 teaspoon Cajun spice mix
- 1/4 teaspoon Old Bay
- 1 egg
- 2 tablespoons dried bread crumbs
- 1 1/2 cups crushed potato chips, for dredging
- 2 tablespoons canola oil, or more for frying

Directions:
- Combine all the ingredients but the potato chips and canola oil.
- Form the mixture into twelve 2 x 1/2-inch round cakes and pat the crushed potato chips on both sides of the crab cakes.
- In a large non-stick skillet over medium heat, heat the oil and sauté the crab cakes for 2 to 3 minutes on each side or until golden and hot throughout.

Marinated Grilled Shrimp

Ingredients:
- 4 cloves garlic, minced
- 1/3 cup extra virgin olive oil
- 1/4 cup tomato sauce
- 2 tablespoons red wine vinegar
- 2 tablespoons chopped fresh basil
- 1/2 teaspoon kosher salt
- 1 teaspoon Old Bay
- 1/4 teaspoon cayenne pepper
- 4 pounds fresh large shrimp, peeled and deveined

metal or wooded skewers (soak in water and olive oil)

Directions:
- In a large bowl, stir together the garlic, olive oil, tomato sauce, and red wine vinegar. Season with basil, salt, Old Bay and cayenne pepper. Add shrimp to the bowl, and stir until evenly coated. Cover, and refrigerate for 30 minutes to 1 hour, stirring once or twice.
- Preheat grill for medium heat. Thread shrimp onto skewers, piercing once near the tail and once near the head. Discard marinade.
- Lightly oil grill grate. Cook shrimp on preheated grill for 2 to 3 minutes per side, or until opaque.

Crabmeat Pinwheels

Makes 10 servings

Ingredients:
- 6 large flour tortillas
- 2 ounces cream cheese, softened
- 1/3 cup mayonnaise
- 2 tablespoons green onions, chopped
- 1/4 cup red bell pepper, chopped
- 1 cup cheddar cheese, shredded
- 1 4 ounce can crabmeat, drained

Directions:
- Combine cream cheese, mayonnaise, onions, red pepper, cheddar cheese and crabmeat. Spread thin layer of mixture on tortillas. Wrap individually in plastic wrap. Chill at least three hours or overnight. When ready to serve, cut into 3/4 inch appetizers.

Shrimp Mold Spread

Ingredients:
- 1 lb shrimp, cubed
- 1 (8 oz) block cream cheese
- 1/2 can of tomato soup
- 1 envelope Knox gelatin
- 1 cup mayonnaise
- 1 cup celery, chopped small
- 3 tablespoon onion, chopped small

Directions:
- Heat tomato soup and add Knox -- stir until dissolved. Pour over cream cheese and mayo - stir till smooth. Add rest of ingredients and pour into mold (LIGHTLY spray it with PAM first).
- Refrigerate for 4 hours or overnight.
- Serve as a spread.

Crab 'n Stuff

Ingredients:
- 8 ounce imitation or real crab meat
- 8 ounce. cream cheese
- Seafood or cocktail sauce

Directions:
- Combine cream cheese and crab. Shape in a ball. Pour seafood sauce over crab ball. Serve

with wheat crackers.

Shrimp with Jalapeno Cheese

Makes 18 servings

Ingredients:
- 2 pounds unpeeled large fresh shrimp
- 6 cups water
- 8 ounces cream cheese, softened
- 2 pickled jalapeno peppers, seeded and finely chopped
- 1 garlic clove, minced
- 2 teaspoons cilantro, freshly chopped
- 1/4 teaspoon salt
- 18 teaspoons pepper

Directions:
- Peel shrimp, leaving tail and first joint of shell intact; cut a deep slit down the length of the outside curve of each shrimp, and devein.
- Bring water to a boil; add shrimp, and cook 3 to 5 minutes or until shrimp turn pink. Drain well; rinse with cold water; chill.
- Combine cream cheese and remaining ingredients; beat well. Fill a decorating bag fitted with metal tip No. 21 with cream cheese mixture. Pipe filling lengthwise into the slits in the shrimp.

Tostaditas with Gulf Crab

Ingredients:
- 1 pound fresh crab meat
- 2 tablespoons mayonnaise
- 2 tablespoons heavy cream
- 1 tablespoon chipotle sauce (optional)
- 1 teaspoon salt
- 3 dozen tortilla rounds or triangles, crisply fried

Directions:
- Carefully check the crab meat for any extraneous pieces of shell. Combine crab meat in a mixing bowl with mayonnaise, heavy cream, salt and chipotle sauce, if desired. Mix until crab is well-coated but do not over mix. Refrigerate until ready to serve.
- Serve on tortilla rounds or triangles with a dollop of guacamole.

Catfish Appetizer

Makes 16 servings

Ingredients:
- 12 ounces cream cheese, softened
- 2 tablespoons mayonnaise
- 2 tablespoons Worcestershire sauce
- 1 tablespoon lemon juice
- Dash of garlic salt
- 1 small onion, finely chopped
- 1/2 cup water
- 1/4 teaspoon salt
- 1 pound catfish fillets
- 1/2 cup chili sauce
- Paprika (optional)

Directions:
- Combine first 5 ingredients; beat at medium speed with electric mixer until smooth. Stir in chopped onion. On a serving platter, spread cream cheese mixture into a 6-inch circle, and pinch up a small rim. Cover and chill at least 3 hours.
- Combine water and salt in a large skillet; bring to a boil, and add fish. Cover, reduce heat, and simmer 10 to 15 minutes or until fish flakes easily with a fork.
- Drain and flake fish with a fork; chill.
- To serve, spoon chili sauce over cream cheese mixture; top with fish. Sprinkle with paprika, if desired.
- Serve with crackers.

Shrimp Cocktail

Ingredients:
- Juice of 1/2 lemon
- 1/2 teaspoon horseradish
- 1/2 teaspoon vinegar
- 8 drops Tabasco sauce
- 1/2 teaspoon tomato catsup

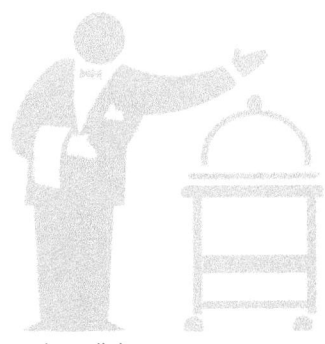

Directions:
- Boil, peel and de-vein shrimp and place them in individual serving dishes.
- Combine above ingredients. This quantity is sufficient for one dish of shrimp. Increase the quantities by the number of dishes you prepare.
- Chill the shrimp in the sauce thoroughly. Serve ice cold.

ASIAN INFLUENCES

Valerie's Asian Pasta Salad

Ingredients:
- 2 bags of shredded cabbage (cole slaw mix)
- 2 packs chicken flavored ramen noodles with seasoning pack
- 5 green onions- thinly chopped
- Shitake mushrooms - thinly sliced (to taste)
- Yellow bell pepper - thinly sliced
- Brocolli - small pieces
- 1/2 cup fresh cilantro - chopped (optional)
- 1/2 cup toasted almond slivers (toast in butter)
- 1/4 cup sunflower seeds
- 1/3 cup canola oil
- 1 tablespoon soy sauce
- 2 tablespoon sugar
- 1 tablespoon balsalmic vinegar
- 1/2 cup rice wine vinegar
- 1/8 teaspoon ground ginger

Directions:
- In a bowl, combine cabbage, green onion, brocolli, bell pepper, cilantro, almonds, and sunflower seeds. Crush noodles and add to the bowl with the seasoning packs and toss.
- In a small bowl, whisk together canola oil, soy sauce, sugar, vinegars, and ginger. Add this dressing no more than 30 minutes prior to serving.
- Place in miniature Chinese take out boxes.

Beef and Pork Wontons

Makes 12 servings

Ingredients:
- 1 egg white
- 1 tablespoon water
- 1 pound lean ground beef
- 1 pound bulk hot Italian sausage
- 1 tablespoon Asian sweet chili sauce, or to taste
- 1 tablespoon Chinese five-spice powder
- 2 teaspoons garlic powder
- 1 green onion, finely chopped
- salt and pepper to taste
- 1 (16 ounce) package wonton wrappers
- 3 cups vegetable oil for frying
- 1/2 cup Asian sweet chili sauce, for dipping

Directions:
- Beat the egg white and water together in a small bowl; set aside. Lightly mix the ground beef, sausage, 1 tablespoon sweet chile sauce, five-spice powder, garlic powder, green onion, and salt and pepper. Place about 1 teaspoonful of the meat mixture onto a wonton wrapper with one corner facing you. Fold in the left and right corners of the wrapper to slightly overlap the filling, then tightly roll the lower corner up to create a pocket around the filling. Continue rolling until just the tip of the remaining corner is visible; brush the corner with the egg white mixture to seal.
- Heat oil in a deep-fryer or large saucepan to 350° F (175° C).
- Fry the egg rolls in the hot oil in batches until golden brown, 3 to 5 minutes. Drain on a paper towel-lined plate. Serve with 1/2 cup of sweet chili sauce.

Valerie's Asian Potstickers

Makes 35-40 servings

Ingredients:
- 1/2 pound ground pork
- 1/4 cup finely chopped scallions
- 2 tablespoons finely chopped red bell pepper
- 1 egg, lightly beaten
- 2 teaspoons ketchup
- 2 teaspoons yellow mustard
- 3 teaspoons Worcestershire sauce
- 2 teaspoons light brown sugar
- 1 1/2 teaspoons kosher salt
- 1 teaspoon freshly ground black pepper
- 1/2 teaspoon cayenne pepper
- 35 to 40 small wonton wrappers
- Water, for sealing wontons
- 3 to 4 tablespoons vegetable oil, for frying
- 1 1/3 cups chicken stock, divided

Directions:
- Preheat oven to 200° F.
- Combine the first 11 ingredients in a medium-size mixing bowl (pork through cayenne). Set aside.
To form the dumplings, remove 1 wonton wrapper from the package, covering the others with a damp cloth. Brush 2 of the edges of the wrapper lightly with water. Place 1/2 rounded teaspoon of the pork mixture in the center of the wrapper. Fold over, seal edges, and shape as desired. Set on a sheet pan and cover with a damp cloth. Repeat procedure until all of the filling is gone.
- Heat a 12-inch saute pan over medium heat. Brush with vegetable oil once hot. Add 8 to 10 potstickers at a time to the pan and cook for 2 minutes, without touching. Once the 2 minutes are up, gently add 1/3 cup chicken stock to the pan, turn the heat down to low, cover, and cook

for another 2 minutes. Remove wontons to a heatproof platter and place in the warm oven. Clean the pan in between batches by pouring in water and allowing the pan to deglaze. Repeat until all the wontons are cooked. Serve immediately.

Tempura Avocado with Shrimp

Ingredients:
- 4 cups canola oil
- 1/2 red onion, diced
- 3 tablespoons minced ginger
- 1 tablespoon minced garlic
- 3/4 pound shrimp, shelled, deveined, cut 1/2-inch pieces
- 3/4 cup thinly sliced bok choy
- 1 cup thinly sliced napa cabbage
- 1/2 red bell pepper, thinly sliced
- 4 tablespoons white wine
- 1 teaspoon sesame oil
- 3 tablespoons soy sauce
- 1 teaspoon black pepper
- 1 teaspoon kosher salt
- 1/2 cup diced green onions
- 2 cups tempura batter
- 4 avocados, large, seeded, skinned
- 1/2 cup sweet chili sauce
- 2 tablespoons black sesame seeds

Directions:
- In a medium saute pan heat 3 tablespoons oil. Add the red onion, ginger, and garlic and saute for 3 minutes. Then add the shrimp, cook for 2 minutes, and then add the bok choy, cabbage, bell peppers. Cook for another 5 minutes to wilt. Deglaze with white wine. Toss in sesame oil, soy sauce, black pepper, salt and green onions. Let mixture cool in a bowl.
- Preheat Dutch oven with oil to 350° F. Mix tempura batter with ice cold water (pancake batter consistency).
- Hollow out 2 tablespoons of avocado from center, add 1/8th of cooled shrimp mixture to cavity of avocado, mixture should sit in avocado securely with only 1/2 to 1/4 of mixture standing out of avocado. Firmly press the mixture into the avocado. Holding the avocado with shrimp mixture, dip entire unit into batter and gently lower into the oil. Cook for 2 to 3 minutes or until golden brown. When cooked, remove and let drain on paper towels, serve hot.
- Drizzle with sweet chili sauce, and sprinkle with black sesame seeds.

Cilantro Wrapped Prawns with Spicy Pickled Pineapple

Makes 24 servings

Ingredients:
Spicy pickled pineapple:
- 2 tablespoons diced red jalapeno
- 2 tablespoons diced white onion
- 6 tablespoons rice wine vinegar
- 1 cup chopped pineapple, without juice
- 2 tablespoons honey
- 1 teaspoon olive oil
- 1 tablespoon lemon juice
- Salt and pepper

Other:
- 12 shrimp (21-25 count) raw, cut lengthwise in 1/2
- Salt and pepper
- 1/2 cup milk
- 1 egg
- 24 wonton skins
- 3 tablespoons minced cilantro leaves
- 1/4 cup julienned red bell pepper

Directions:
- For the spicy pickled pineapple: In a medium saute pan, heat oil, add pepper and onions, lightly saute, Combine all ingredients, heat for 3 minutes on medium heat and let cool for 1 hour.
- Season shrimp with salt and pepper. Mix milk and egg, dredge wonton wrapper in milk, then add 1/2 piece shrimp to corner of wrapper, add a pinch of cilantro, and 1 piece of red bell pepper, roll up, and place seam side down in medium pan with canola oil on medium to high heat. Fry until light brown.

Bacon Wrapped Water Chestnuts

Makes 16 servings

Ingredients:
- 16 fresh water chestnuts
- 1/3 cup soy sauce
- 1/3 cup brown sugar, or as needed
- 8 slices raw bacon, cut in half
- 16 toothpicks

Directions:
- Peel and rinse the fresh water chestnuts (if using canned water chestnuts, rinse in warm run-

ning water and drain).
- Soak the water chestnuts in the soy sauce for 2 1/2 hours.
- Preheat the oven to 350° F. Remove the water chestnuts from the soy sauce and roll in the brown sugar. Wrap a piece of cut bacon around the water chestnut and secure with a toothpick.
- Place the water chestnuts on a rack in a shallow pan. Bake for 30 minutes, turning them over once. Alternately, they can be broiled for 5-6 minutes.
- The appetizers can be prepared ahead of time and frozen before cooking. Placed in a sealed bag in the freezer, they should last for 2-3 months.

Paper Wrapped Chicken

Makes 24 servings

Ingredients:
- 2 pounds boneless, skinless chicken breasts

Marinade:
- 3 tablespoons soy sauce
- 3 tablespoons oyster sauce
- 1 slice ginger, shredded
- 1 tablespoon sesame oil
- 1 tablespoon sherry
- 3 teaspoons sugar
- 1/2 teaspoon five spice powder

Other:
- 3-4 Chinese dried mushrooms, softened and thinly sliced (24 slices, 1 for each packet)
- 3 green onions, thinly sliced on the diagonal (2-3 slices for each packet)
- 24 sprigs cilantro (coriander leaves)
- 24 6 inch squares of cellophane paper, cooking parchment paper, or aluminum foil
- Peanut oil for deep-frying

Directions:
- Cut the chicken into thin slices roughly 2 1/2 inches long (to make 48 slices). Pound lightly on the back of the chicken to tenderize.
- Combine the marinade ingredients. Add the chicken. Cover and marinate in the refrigerator for 45 minutes. Add the mushrooms and green onions and marinate for another 15 minutes. (This allows the vegetables to absorb the marinade).
- To wrap the chicken: paper-wrapped chicken is normally wrapped envelope style. Take a square of paper and lay it out in front of you. Add 2 of the chicken slices, 1 slice of mushroom, 2 slices of green onion and a coriander sprig (if desired) in the middle, being sure to keep the filling in the center and not near the edges. Bring the bottom flap up over the chicken. Fold the right side over toward the middle, then the left side, so that one is overlapping the other. Fold the top flap down, tucking it inside the opening to seal the package. It is very important to make sure the packets are well sealed so that no oil seeps in.

- Heat wok and add oil for deep-frying. When the oil is ready, slide the packages in, about 6 at a time so as not to overcrowd the wok. Deep-fry the packets, stirring occasionally, until the chicken is cooked through (about 3 minutes). Drain on paper towels. Continue deep-frying the rest of the packets.
- Serve the chicken packets on a large platter, garnished with greens if desired. Guests can open the packets with either chopsticks or their fingers.
- This recipe can be prepared ahead up to the deep-frying or baking stage and refrigerated or frozen. Bring back to room temperature before cooking.

Asian Lettuce Wraps

Makes 4 servings

Ingredients:
- 2 teaspoons vegetable oil
- 1 pound ground beef
- 2 inch piece ginger, peeled and finely grated
- 2 scallions, chopped
- 2 cloves garlic, minced
- 2 tablespoons soy sauce
- 1 teaspoon red pepper flakes
- 1/4 cup hoisin sauce
- 1/4 cup chopped peanuts
- Salt and freshly ground black pepper

Directions:
- 1 head Boston lettuce, leaves separated, cleaned and dried In a skillet over medium-high heat, add the vegetable oil and saute beef until brown.
- Stir in ginger, scallions, garlic, soy sauce, red pepper flakes, and hoisin and cook for 1 minute. Remove from the heat and stir in the peanuts. Season with salt and pepper and serve warm wrapped in lettuce cups.

Asian Pork Shui Mai

Makes 15 servings

Ingredients:
- 1 pound ground pork
- 1 cup finely chopped water chestnuts
- 1 tablespoon soy sauce
- 1 tablespoon rice wine vinegar
- 1 tablespoon sesame oil
- 2 teaspoons sugar
- 2 teaspoons freshly grated ginger

- 2 tablespoons cornstarch
- 1 teaspoon coarse salt
- 1/2 teaspoon finely ground black pepper
- 30 wonton wrappers

Dipping Sauce:
- 1/2 cup soy sauce
- 2 tablespoons black vinegar, or rice wine vinegar
- 1 teaspoon Oriental red chile paste
- 1/2 teaspoon sugar
- 1 tablespoon minced garlic

Directions:
- Combine the pork, water chestnuts, soy sauce, vinegar, oil, sugar, ginger, cornstarch, salt and pepper in a bowl and mix well to combine (hands work well for this).
- Place a dumpling wrapper in the palm of one hand and cup it loosely. Place a generous tablespoon of filling in the center of the wrapper.
- With your free hand, gather the sides of the wrapper around the filling, letting the wrapper pleat naturally. Squeeze the middle gently and tap the dumpling to flatten the bottom so that it can stand upright. The meat filling will show a little at the top. Make the remaining dumplings in the same manner.
- Arrange filled dumplings about 1/4 inch apart in two steamer trays that have been lined with wet cheesecloth. (At this point, you can refrigerate dumplings, covered, for 24 hours.)
- When ready to steam, fill a wok or lower part of a steamer with water so that it comes within an inch of the steamer tray, and bring to a rolling boil. Stack the steamer trays in the wok or steamer, cover tightly, and steam dumplings for 25 minutes over high heat, reversing the trays after 10 minutes.
- Use a slotted spoon to transfer dumplings to a platter and serve with spicy dipping sauce.
- For Dipping Sauce: Combine ingredients in a small bowl and serve with pork dumplings.

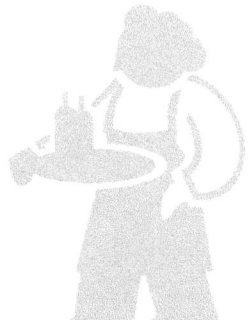
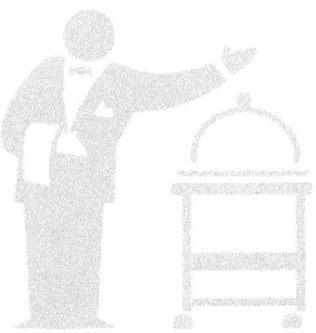

MEATLESS
PARTY SOLUTIONS

Spanikopita

Makes 15 Servings

Ingredients:

- 2 (10 ounce) packages frozen chopped spinach, thawed and well drained
- 1/2 cup crumbled feta cheese
- 1/2 cup shredded mozzarella cheese
- 1/2 cup grated Parmesan cheese
- 1 clove garlic, minced
- 1/2 teaspoon salt
- 1 (16 ounce) package whole wheat phyllo dough
- 1/2 cup unsalted butter, melted

Directions:
- Preheat an oven to 375° F (190° C). Lightly grease a baking sheet. Mix the spinach, feta cheese, mozzarella cheese, Parmesan cheese, garlic, and salt in a bowl.
- Arrange one sheet of phyllo dough on a clean work surface and brush with melted butter. Cover the remaining phyllo dough with a damp towel. Place a second sheet of phyllo on top and brush with butter, then place a third sheet on top. Cut the buttered phyllo lengthwise into four strips.
- Place about 1 tablespoon of the spinach mixture on the bottom of each strip. Take the bottom right corner and fold the dough over the filling to make a triangle. Fold the bottom left corner up to make another triangle. Continue folding until all the dough is folded. Arrange the stuffed triangles, seam-side down, on the prepared baking sheet. Lightly brush the triangle with butter. Repeat with the remaining phyllo dough and spinach filling.
- Bake in the preheated oven until golden brown, about 20 minutes. Cool slightly before serving.

Caprese on a Stick

Makes 20 servings

Ingredients:
- 5 cups cherry tomatoes, halved
- 2 1/2 (.6 ounce) packages fresh basil leaves
- 2 1/2 (16 ounce) packages small fresh mozzarella balls
- Toothpicks
- 1/3 cup and 2 tablespoons olive oil
- Salt and pepper (to taste)

Directions:
- Thread a tomato half, a small piece of basil leaf, and a mozzarella ball onto toothpicks until all ingredients are used. Drizzle the olive oil over the tomato, cheese and basil, leaving the end of

the toothpick clean. Sprinkle with salt and pepper. Serve immediately.

South African Spicy Potato Noodles

Makes 15 servings

Ingredients
Green Chile Paste:
- 1/3 cup and 2 tablespoons chopped fresh green chile peppers
- 1 tablespoon and 2-1/2 teaspoons coarsely chopped garlic
- 3 tablespoons and 2-1/4 teaspoons fresh ginger, peeled and coarsely chopped
- 1 3/4 teaspoons salt
- 1/4 teaspoon ground turmeric
- 1 tablespoon and 3/4 teaspoon vegetable oil

Noodles:
- 2 pounds potatoes, peeled
- 5 2/3 cups water
- 7 cups chickpea flour
- 1 tablespoon and 1 3/4 teaspoons salt
- 1 3/4 teaspoons ground turmeric
- 3 tablespoons and 2 1/4 teaspoons mustard oil
- Canola oil for deep frying

Directions:
- Combine the chiles, garlic, ginger, 1 teaspoon salt, 1/8 teaspoon turmeric, and 2 teaspoons vegetable oil in a food processor or mortar and pestle and process into a fine paste. (Add a tablespoon of water if you need more liquid.) Set aside.
- Place the potatoes in a saucepan with the water and bring to a boil over high heat. Reduce the heat to low, cover the pan, and cook the potatoes until they're soft and easily pierced with a fork, about 15 minutes. Reserve the cooking water.
- Mash the potatoes while they're still warm, using some of the cooking water to get a smooth consistency. Mix in 1 tablespoon green chile paste, chickpea flour, 2 1/2 teaspoons salt, 1 teaspoon turmeric, and mustard oil. Add enough reserved potato-cooking water as needed to make a soft dough. Taste the dough for heat level and seasoning (the dough will taste raw, but should be salty and spicy; the flavors will mellow slightly during cooking). Add more salt and chile paste if desired.
- Heat the cooking oil in a deep pan over medium-high heat. Use a potato ricer (or sev machine, if you have one) to press noodles into the oil. Fry until golden brown and crisp, about two minutes. Use a skimmer or slotted spoon to transfer the noodles to a paper towel-lined bowl. Repeat until all noodles are fried. Store in an airtight container for up to two weeks.

Double Tomato Bruchetta

Makes 12 servings

Ingredients:
- 6 roma (plum) tomatoes, chopped
- 1/2 cup sun-dried tomatoes, packed in oil
- 3 cloves minced garlic
- 1/4 cup olive oil
- 2 tablespoons balsamic vinegar
- 1/4 cup fresh basil, stems removed
- 1/4 teaspoon salt
- 1/4 teaspoon ground black pepper
- 1 French baguette
- 2 cups shredded mozzarella cheese

Directions:
- Preheat the oven on broiler setting.
- In a large bowl, combine the roma tomatoes, sun-dried tomatoes, garlic, olive oil, vinegar, basil, salt, and pepper. Allow the mixture to sit for 10 minutes.
- Cut the baguette into 3/4-inch slices. On a baking sheet, arrange the baguette slices in a single layer. Broil for 1 to 2 minutes, until slightly brown.
- Divide the tomato mixture evenly over the baguette slices. Top the slices with mozzarella cheese.
- Broil for 5 minutes, or until the cheese is melted.

Spicy Bean Salsa

Makes 12 servings

Ingredients:
- 1 (15 ounce) can black-eyed peas
- 1 (15 ounce) can black beans, rinsed and drained
- 1 (15 ounce) can whole kernel corn, drained
- 1/2 cup chopped onion
- 1/2 cup chopped green bell pepper
- 1 (4 ounce) can diced jalapeno peppers
- 1 (14.5 ounce) can diced tomatoes, drained
- 1 cup Italian-style salad dressing
- 1/2 teaspoon garlic salt

Directions:
- In a medium bowl, combine black-eyed peas, black beans, corn, onion, green bell pepper, jalapeno peppers and tomatoes. Season with Italian-style salad dressing and garlic salt; mix well.

Cover, and refrigerate overnight to blend flavors.

Avocado Feta Salsa

Makes 12 servings

Ingredients:
- 2 plum tomatoes, chopped
- 1 ripe avocado - peeled, pitted and chopped
- 1/4 cup finely chopped red onion
- 1 clove garlic, minced
- 1 tablespoon snipped fresh parsley
- 1 tablespoon chopped fresh oregano
- 1 tablespoon olive oil
- 1 tablespoon red or white wine vinegar
- 4 ounces crumbled feta cheese

Directions:
- In a bowl, gently stir together tomatoes, avocados, onion, and garlic. Mix in parsley and oregano. Gently stir in olive oil and vinegar. Then stir in feta. Cover, and chill for 2 to 6 hours.

Artichoke and Roasted Red Pepper Dip

Makes 24 servings

Ingredients:
- 2 tablespoons butter
- 1 leek, diced
- 2 (6.5 ounce) jars marinated artichoke hearts, drained and chopped
- 1 (7 ounce) jar roasted red peppers, drained and chopped
- 3/4 cup freshly grated Parmesan cheese
- 3 tablespoons mayonnaise

Directions:
- Preheat oven to 350° F (175° C).
- Melt butter in a saucepan over medium heat. Saute diced leek until tender. Stir in the artichoke hearts, roasted red peppers, Parmesan cheese, and mayonnaise. Transfer to an 8x8 inch baking dish.
- Bake for 30 minutes in the preheated oven, or until bubbly and lightly browned.

Fresh Tortilla Triangles

Makes 32 servings

Ingredients
- 2 cups canola or other vegetable oil
- 8 (6 inch) corn tortillas, quartered
- Salt (to taste)

Directions
- Heat oil in a 10-inch skillet to 370 °. Drop triangles in hot oil, 8 at a time. Fry, turning chips once or twice, until they stop sizzling and turn golden brown, about 2 minutes. Remove with tongs or a slotted spoon and drain on a wire rack set over a shallow pan. Sprinkle with salt immediately.

Edamame Hummus

Makes 3 cups

Ingredients:
- 1/2 pound frozen shelled edamame (green soy beans), about 1 1/2 cups
- 1/4 cup Tahini (seasame seed paste)
- 1/4 cup water
- 1/2 teaspoon freshly-grated lemon zest
- 3 tablespoons fresh-squeezed lemon juice
- 2 cloves garlic, smashed
- 3/4 teaspoon coarse salt
- 1/2 teaspoon ground cumin
- 1/4 teaspoon ground coriander
- 3 tablespoons extra-virgin olive oil, divided
- 1 tablespoon chopped fresh flat-leaf parsley

Directions:
- Boil the beans in salted water for 4 to 5 minutes, or microwave, covered, for 2 to 3 minutes.
- In a food processor, puree the edamame, tahini, water, lemon zest, lemon juice, garlic, salt, cumin, and coriander until smooth. With the motor running, slowly drizzle in 2 tablespoons of the olive oil and mix until absorbed.
- Transfer to a small bowl, stir in the parsley and drizzle with remaining oil 1 tablespoon of olive oil. You can also garnish with some sesame seeds.
- Serve with fresh vegetables or pita bread.

Hot Garlic-Parmesan Soufflé

Ingredients:
- 15 cloves garlic, peeled
- 2 cups chicken broth or stock
- 2 (8 ounce) packages cream cheese, room temperature
- 1 cup freshly-grated parmesan cheese
- 1 (10.5 ounce) can cream of mushroom soup, undiluted
- 2 egg yolks, beaten
- 1 loaf baguette bread, thinly sliced.

Directions:
- Preheat oven to 350° F.
- In a medium saucepan over medium-high heat, combine garlic cloves and chicken broth; bring to a boil and poach 15 minutes or until garlic is soft. Remove garlic cloves to a small bowl and allow them to cool. When cool, mash with a fork; set aside.
- Cook and reduce chicken broth to a glaze; remove from heat and set aside.
- In a large bowl, combine cream cheese, parmesan cheese, mushroom soup, garlic-chicken glaze, mashed garlic, and egg yolks; stir until well blended. Transfer into a shallow ungreased 1 1/2-quart soufflé dish.
- Bake, uncovered, 45 to 50 minutes or until golden brown. Remove from oven and serve with bread.

Grilled Figs with Goat Cheese and Honey

Ingredients:
- 12 fresh figs
- 1 small package of mild goat cheese
- 12 grape leaves (bottled grape leaves), drained and rinsed*
- Honey

Directions:

*To use fresh grape leaves: Grape leaves are best picked from grape vines in the spring, while they are still tender. Select young whole, medium leaves. Note: Be sure and pick them before the first spray as some sprays are toxic. Most of the spays used today are non-toxic and water soluble, but sulfur taste is not what you want on your grapes. Pick approximately 1 1/2 pounds of fresh leaves which are the same as one jar of preserved leaves. Using scissors, cut off the stems and either soak in very hot water for 15 minutes to soften or blanch grape leaves until they are soft (the time will depend on the leaves - fresh ones will only take a minute) They can be washed and frozen between layers of waxed paper or plastic wrap and will keep for a year.
- Remove stems from figs. Using a small sharp knife open up the fig from the top to about the middle with an X-cut. Place a small amount of goat's cheese into the opening. NOTE: Fill figs with goat cheese by squeezing a small amount of cheese into the bottom of each fig. The figs will plump up when filled.

- Wrap each fig with a grape leaf and skewer 2 to 3 figs on each skewer.
- Place fig skewers on a hot grill and cook for approximately 2 to 3 minutes, turning once. Remove from grill; drizzle with honey before serving.

Green Bean Pate

Makes 2 cups

Ingredients:
- 1/2 pound fresh green beans, ends trimmed
- 3 large onions, peeled and sliced
- 1/4 cup vegetable broth
- 3 hard-cooked egg whites
- 1 cup walnut or pecan pieces
- 1 teaspoon kosher salt or to taste
- 1 teaspoon coarsely-ground black pepper
- Assorted crackers

Directions:
- In a large saucepan over medium-high heat, cook green beans in water for 12 minutes. Remove from heat and drain. In a medium frying pan over medium heat, sauté onions in vegetable broth 30 minutes or until onions are well done, stirring frequently. Remove from heat.
- In a food processor, place green beans, onions, hard-cooked eggs whites, walnuts or pecans, salt and pepper; whirl until a pate-like consistency is reached. Transfer into a serving bowl and serve with assorted crackers.

Spanish Tomato Toast (Pan con Tomate)

Makes 8 servings

Ingredients:
- 8 slices sourdough or country-style bread, cut into 3/4 inch thick slices
- 4 cloves garlic peeled and cut in half
- 4 small ripe tomatoes cut in half*
- Cruet of extra-virgin olive oil
- Small bowl of coarse salt or sea salt
- Freshly ground peppercorns

Directions:
*For the best flavor, use vine-ripe tomatoes, preferably home grown ones.
- Grill the bread approximately 2 to 4 minutes per side on a grill or toast it lightly in the oven.
- Once the bread is toasted, rub 1/2 clove of garlic, cut side of half, over the bread while still warm.

(continued)

- Use a fresh piece of garlic for each slice. Rub tomato (cut side) over the bread, pressing firmly to push the pulp into the bread, until the toast is covered with tomato; discard the skins and remaining pulp. Drizzle olive oil over the bread and tomatoes; sprinkle with salt and a couple grind of pepper. Serve immediately.

There are two ways to serve tomato bread:
- The first is for the cook to do the rubbing and drizzling.
- The second is to provide each person with a clove of garlic, half tomato, cruet of oil, and bowl of salt and let him or her do the work. The second way is more fun.

Optional garnish, choose one or a combination:
- 1/2 cup green Spanish olives
- 12 anchovy fillets, soaked in cold water for 10 minutes, drained, and patted dry
- 6 paper-thin slices Spanish ham or prosciutto
- 12 paper-thin slices Manchego

Black Truffle Canapes

Makes 20 canapes

Ingredients:
- 5 thin slices firm, white sandwich bread
- 2 tablespoons unsalted butter, melted
- 7 ounces prepared pate with truffles*
- 2 to 3 tablespoons crème fraiche or sour cream
- Black truffle shavings

*Can substitute any good-quality pate.

Directions:
- Preheat oven to 350° F.
- Brush bread with melted butter and cut out approximately twenty (20) 1 1/2- to 2 inch circles with round cookie cutter; arrange, buttered sides up, on a large baking sheet. Bake in middle of oven approximately 7 to 10 minutes or until pale golden. Remove from oven and cool completely. Note: Toasts may be made 1 day ahead and kept in an airtight container at room temperature.
- To prepare, place thin slices of pate on each toast round. Top with crème fraiche or sour cream and truffle shavings. Note: You always want to maximize the truffle flavor, using the least amount of the ingredient as possible. So always slice into paper-thin wedges or strips. Use a truffle shaver (similar to a cheese grater) when shaving truffles.
- Cover with plastic wrap until ready to serve, but don't let sit too long as bread toasts will become soft.

SWEET TREATS

Banana Bisque with Cinnamon Croutons

Ingredients:
- Cinnamon Croutons - see recipe below
- 3 cups peeled and sliced ripe bananas (about 4 large bananas)
- 3 cups half-and-half cream
- 1/2 teaspoon ground cinnamon

Directions:
- Prepare Cinnamon Croutons; set aside and let cool.
- In a food processor or blender, place sliced bananas and cream; process until smooth. Add the cinnamon and the blend the mixture again.
- Refrigerate the soup until well chilled.
- Serve in small glass bowl with Cinnamon Croutons.

Cinnamon Croutons

Ingredients:
- 1 loaf two-day old French bread
- 6 tablespoons butter, melted

Directions:
- Preheat oven to 400° F.
- Remove crusts from the loaf of bread and cut into 1/2-inch thick slices. Cut the slices into small cubes. Brush the cubes of bread with melted butter and bake them on a baking sheet until they are golden, approximately 10 minutes. Remove from oven. While the croutons are still hot, sprinkle them lightly with the ground cinnamon. Let croutons cool completely before using in the bisque.

Honeydew Melon, Mint & Green Grape Toothpick Appetizer

Ingredients:
- Honeydew melon
- Fresh mint leaves
- Green grapes
- Toothpicks

Directions:
- Cut melon into 1/2-inch pieces, thread on toothpicks with mint leaves and grapes, serve on a platter.

Sweet Weiners

Ingredients:
- 1 package cocktail weenies
- 1 jar barbeque sauce
- 3 tablespoons grape jelly

Directions:
- Place weenies in a crock pot with enough barbeque sauce to liberally coat, then add grape jelly.

French Chocolate Truffles

Ingredients:
- 24 ounces semi-sweet dark chocolate, cut in small pieces
- 14 ounce can sweetened condensed milk
- 2 cups pecan nuts, toasted, finely ground
- 2 teaspoons vanilla
- Dash of kosher salt

Coat Truffles in:
- Sprinkles
- Shredded coconut
- Pecans, finely chopped
- Cocoa powder

Directions:
- Melt semi-sweet dark chocolate in a saucepan over low heat stirring constantly, do not burn. Remove from heat, stir in sweetened condensed milk, pecan nuts, vanilla and salt. Cool 5 minutes.
- Using your hands roll into walnut sized balls; coat with sprinkles or shredded coconut or finely chopped pecans or roll in cocoa powder. Place truffles single layer on a sheet pan, cover and refrigerate until set.

White Chocolate Pretzels

Makes 12 servings

Ingredients:
- 1/2 cup pretzel sticks
- 1/2 cup salted peanuts
- 1/2 cup crisp rice cereal
- 4 (1 ounce) squares white baking chocolate
- 1 teaspoon shortening

Directions:
- In a bowl, combine the pretzels, peanuts and cereal. In a microwave or heavy saucepan, melt chocolate and shortening, stir until smooth. Pour over pretzel mixture; toss to coat evenly. Drop by heaping tablespoonfuls onto waxed paper; cool.

Cinnamon Popcorn

Makes 16 servings

Ingredients:
- 4 quarts popped popcorn
- 1 cup butter or margarine
- 2/3 cup sugar
- 1 tablespoon cinnamon

Directions:
- Place popcorn in a large bowl. In a microwave-safe bowl, combine the butter, sugar and cinnamon. Microwave on high for 1 minute; stir. Microwave 1 minute longer or until the butter is melted. Pour over popcorn and toss to coat. Transfer to two greased 15 x 10 x 1 inch baking pans. Bake, uncovered, at 300° F for 10 minutes. Cool. Store in an airtight container.

Praline Pecans

Makes 12 servings

Ingredients:
- 1 cup sugar
- 1 cup packed brown sugar
- 1/2 cup water
- 2 tablespoons honey
- 1/2 teaspoon ground cinnamon
- 3 teaspoons vanilla extract
- 1/4 teaspoon rum extract
- 3 cups pecan halves

Directions:
- In a heavy saucepan, combine the sugars, water, honey and cinnamon. Bring to a boil over medium heat; do not stir. Cook over medium heat until a candy thermometer reads 240° F (soft-ball stage). Remove from the heat; add extracts. Cool to lukewarm without stirring.
- Beat with a mixer for 2-3 minutes or until creamy. Stir in pecans until coated. Turn onto waxed paper (mixture will be sticky); separate large clumps. Cool for several hours or until dry and sugary. Store in an airtight container.

Sweet Potato Balls

Makes 18 servings

Ingredients:
- 5 pounds canned sweet potatoes
- 1/2 cup butter
- 2 pinches salt (optional)
- 6 cups crushed cornflakes cereal
- 1 1/2 cups real maple syrup
- 20 large marshmallows

Directions:
- Drain sweet potatoes and put into large mixing bowl. Mash the potatoes with butter or margarine. Salt to taste.
- Hand pat mixture into 3 inch diameter balls. Roll in crushed corn flakes and put into 9 x 12 inch greased baking dish. Pour maple syrup evenly over all balls.
- Bake at 325° F (165° C) for 40 minutes. The last fifteen minutes put a marshmallow over each ball.

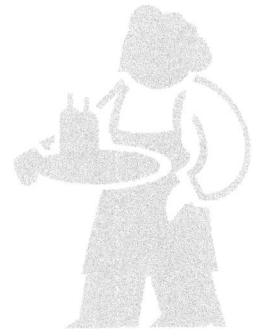

DRINKS & PUNCHES

Pomegranate Margarita

Makes 12 servings

Ingredients:
- 2 cups tequila
- 2 cups triple sec
- 1/2 cup confectioners' sugar
- 8 cups ice
- 2 cups pomegranate juice
- 2 cups fresh lime juice

Directions:
- Pour the tequila and triple sec into a pitcher. Sprinkle in the confectioners' sugar, and stir to dissolve. Add the ice, and pour in the pomegranate juice and lime juice. Stir to mix, then serve. You can add more tequila to taste if you're a professional.

Caribbean Martini

Makes 12 servings

Ingredients:
- 24 ounce Bacardi® Limon rum
- 12 ounce Cointreau® orange liqueur
- 12 ounce Blue Curacao liqueur

Directions:
- Combine the Bacardi Limon rum, Cointreau, and blue Curacao in a shaker with ice. Shake and strain into chilled cocktail glass. Garnish with an orange twist, and serve.

Kiwi Margarita

Makes 12 servings

Ingredients:
- 1 1/2 cups superfine sugar
- 1 cup gold tequila
- 1 cup triple sec
- 6 large kiwis, peeled
- 3 cups fresh lime juice
- 6 cups small ice cubes

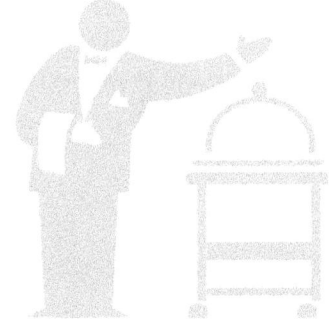

Directions:
- Combine the sugar, tequila, triple sec, kiwis, and lime juice in a blender; fill with ice cubes;

blend until smooth.

JELLO Shots - Malibu Islands

Ingredients:
- 1 package JELLO (Island Pineapple)
- 1 part Malibu Rum

Directions:
- Add JELLO to boiling water and substitute cold water with Malibu rum. Pour into shot glasses and refrigerate for 4 hrs.

JELLO Shots - Wild Berry

Ingredients:
- 1 package JELLO (Wildberry)
- Gordon's Wildberry Vodka

Directions:
- Add JELLO to boiling water and substitute cold water with vodka or water and vodka (depending on how strong you want them you can go full strength or half and half). Pour into shot glasses or small paper cups.

Champagne Punch

Ingredients:
- 3 cups champagne (chilled)
- 2 cups sparkling water (chilled)
- 1/2 cup Brandy
- 1/2 cup Cointreau

Directions:
- Combine all of the ingredients and serve in punch cups.

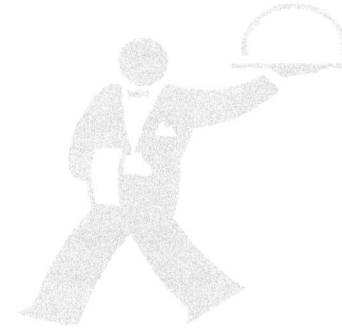

Love Juice

Ingredients:
- 3 cans beer (12 ounce cans)
- 3 lemons - sliced
- 3 limes - sliced
- 2 cans fruit punch (frouncesen concentrate)
- 1/5 gallon Vodka

Directions:
- Put 5 pounds of ice in a cooler and dig a well in the middle of the ice. Pour the frouncesen

concentrate in the well, add the vodka and the beer. Mix well then add the chopped fruit. Cover and let stand for 15 minutes, then stir and serve in punch cups.

Mojito Diablo

Makes 12 servings

Ingredients:
- 18 ounces white tequila
- 6 ounces creme de cassis
- 24 lime wedges
- 144 fresh mint leaves
- 54 ounces 7-Up® soda
- 12 tablespoons brown sugar

Directions:
- Muddle sugar, mint and squeezed lime wedges in mixing tin until mixture smells like spearmint gum. Fill with ice, add tequila and cassis, shake until the tin is icey to the touch. Pour into a collins glass, top with 7-Up and garnish with a sugarcane stick and fresh mint.

Apple Mojito

Makes 12 servings

- 24 ounces Bacardi® Big Apple rum
- 72 ounces club soda
- 36 lime wedges
- 24 teaspoons sugar
- 36 fresh mint sprigs

Directions:
- Add the lime, sugar and mint sprigs to a highball glass and muddle with a muddler. Add several ice cubes and pour in the Bacardi apple rum. Top with club soda (adjust to taste), and stir. Garnish with an apple slice and a lime wedge, and serve.

Passion Fruit Mojito

Makes 12 servings

Ingredients:
- 900 milliliters Havana Club® dark rum (3 years old)
- 12 teaspoons (heaped) Muscovado sugar
- 72 lime wedges
- 132 mint leaves

- 300 milliliters passion-fruit puree
- 600 milliliters soda
- 2/3 of a glass crushed ice

Directions:
- Crush well the lime, sugar, soda, 8 to 10 limes' leaves and a teaspoon of crushed ice, then add ice, passion fruit and rum, mix vigorously for one minute, and garnish with rest of mint and a straw.

Valerie's Fruit Cocktail

Makes 12 servings

Ingredients:
- 6 ounces Absolut® Mandrin vodka
- 6 ounces Captain Morgan® Parrot Bay pineapple rum
- 6 ounces peach schnapps
- 6 ounces Midori® melon liqueur
- 6 ounces DeKuyper® Sour Apple Pucker schnapps
- 12 splash pineapple juice
- 12 splash grenadine syrup

Directions:
- Combine all ingredients in a cocktail shaker half-filled with ice cubes. Shake well and strain into an old-fashioned glass half-filled with ice cubes. Serve.

Jessica's Cosmopolitan

Makes 12 servings

Ingredients:
- 15 ounces Absolut® Citron vodka
- 3 ounces lime juice
- 3 ounces triple sec
- 3 cups cranberry juice

Directions:
- Combine all ingredients in a cocktail shaker with ice. Shake briefly and pour into a chilled cocktail glass. Garnish with a lime twist.

Raspberry Cosmopolitan

Makes 12 servings

Ingredients:
- 24 ounces Stolichnaya® raspberry vodka
- 7.92 ounces triple sec
- 12 ounces cranberry juice
- 6 ounces lime juice

Directions:
- Shake with ice, strain into a chilled cocktail glass, and serve.

Terry's Caribbean Cosmopolitan

Makes 12 servings

Ingredients:
- 18 ounces Bacardi® Limon rum
- 12 ounces cranberry juice
- 12 ounces Cointreau® orange liqueur
- 6 ounces fresh lime juice

Directions:
- Shake all ingredients with ice and strain into a chilled martini glass. Garnish with flamed orange peel, and serve.

7-Up Punch

Makes 12 servings

Ingredients:
- 8 cinnamon sticks
- 6 cups sugar
- 24 cups water
- 36 cups orange juice
- 3 cups lemon juice
- 12 cups pineapple juice
- 24 liters 7-Up® soda

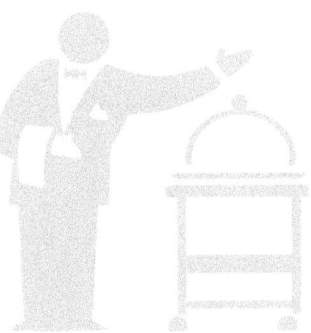

Directions:
- In a sauce pan simmer cinnamon sticks with water and sugar about 5 minutes. Cool. In a large bowl, combine cinnamon mixture with orange juice, lemon juice, and pineapple juice. Pour in 7-Up just before serving.

Apple Cider Punch

Makes 12 servings

Ingredients:
- 48 quarts apple cider
- 12 cup packed brown sugar
- 72 ounces frouncesen lemonade
- 72 ounces frouncesen orange juice
- 72 whole cloves
- 72 whole allspice
- 12 teaspoons ground nutmeg
- 36 cinnamon sticks

Directions:
- If you use the whole all spice and cloves, tie them in cheesecloth. Heat the mixture. Stir occasionally. If you want an alcoholic drink, rum would be nice.

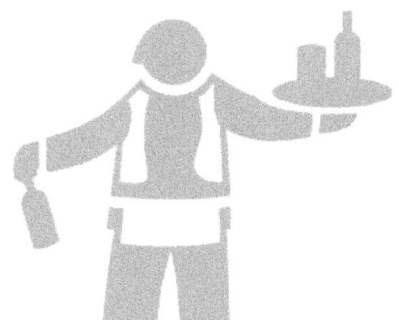
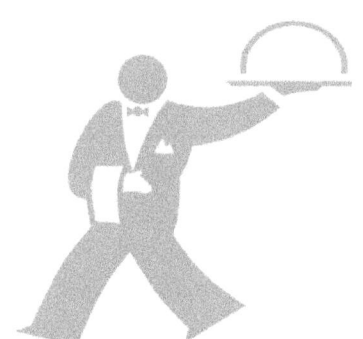

INDEX

Symbols

7-Up Punch 89

A

Alaskan Spicy Spinach Dip 15
Apple Cider Punch 90
Apple Gouda Quesadillas 13
Apple Mojito 87
Artichoke and Roasted Red Pepper Dip 74
Asian Lettuce Wraps 68
Asian Pork Shui Mai 68
Avocado Feta Salsa 74
Avocado Mango Salsa 6

B

Baba Ganouj 26
Bacon Olive Wraps 17
Bacon Wrapped Water Chestnuts 66
Baked Cream Cheese Wontons 30
Banana Bisque with Cinnamon Croutons 80
Beef and Pork Wontons 63
Beef Spring Rolls with Carrots and Cilantro 45
Beefy Cheese Ball 50
Black Truffle Canapes 78
Brazilian Onion Bites 6
Buffalo Chicken Dip 37
Buttery Blue Cheese Spread with Walnuts 27

C

Cajun Deviled Eggs 22
Caprese on a Stick 71
Caribbean Fruity Salsa 18
Caribbean Martini 85
Catfish Appetizer 61
Catfish Mini Cakes 55
Ceviche 54
Champagne Punch 86
Cheese Ball Pastry 32
Cheese Triangles 34
Chicken and Sun-Dried Tomato Bruschetta 14
Chicken Satay Appetizers 37
Chili Chicken Strips 38, 39
Chocolate Cheese Cake Dip 26
Chocolate Covered Strawberries 11
Cilantro Wrapped Prawns with Spicy Pickled Pineapple 66
Cinnamon Croutons 80
Cinnamon Popcorn 82
Cocktail Meatballs 46
Coffee Flavored Fruit Dip 12
Corned Beef Bagel Dip 49
Corned Beef Party Puffs 49
Crab Cake Bites 52
Crabmeat Pinwheels 59
Crab 'n Stuff 59

D

Double Tomato Bruchetta 73
Double Tomato Bruschetta 14

E

Edamame Hummus 75

F

Fig Appetizers with Goat Cheese and Almonds 5
French Chocolate Truffles 81
French Onion Quiche Appetizers 7
Fresh Tortilla Triangles 74
Fruit Dip 12
Fruit Guacamole 10

G

Gingered Mango Salsa 10
Gougeres 35
Grape and Avocado Salsa 5
Greek Style Avocado Dip 10
Green Bean Pate 77
Grilled Figs with Goat Cheese and Honey 76
Grilled Fruit Sates 13
Grilled Sirloin Kabobs 48
Guacamole Deviled Eggs 23

H

Herb and Cheese Mini Quiche 34
Herbed Shrimp On Grits Cakes 52
Honeydew Melon, Mint & Green Grape Toothpick Appetizer 80
Honey Mustard Drummettes 40
Hot Artichoke Dip 32
Hot Garlic-Parmesan Soufflé 75

J

Jalapeno Hummus 11
Jalapeno Jelly Cheese Loaf 27
Jalapeno Sausage Poppers 33
Jamaican Meat Patties 43
Java Style Beef Sate 45
Jazzed Up Olives 3
JELLO Shots - Malibu Islands 86
JELLO Shots - Wild Berry 86
Jessica's Cosmopolitan 88

K

Kiwi Margarita 85

L

Leftover Salmon Patties 56
Lime & Honey Pears 5
Lobster Fritters 56
Love Juice 86

M

Mandarin Chicken Bites 40
Marinated Grilled Shrimp 58
Marinated Mushrooms & Artichokes

INDEX

Maryland Crab Dipping Sauce 53
Mexican Beef Egg Rolls 44
Mexican Layered Dip 12
Mini Blinis with Caviar 54
Mississippi Caliente Caviar 18
Mojito Diablo 87
Muffin Pan Crab Cakes 57
Mushroom Appetizers 4

O

Olive Pecan Spread 17
Onion Bhaji 7
Onion Brie Appetizers 8
Onion Jam Appetizer On Toast Points 9
Orange and Rosemary Baked Olives 16
Orange Glazed Cocktail Sausages 43

P

Paper Wrapped Chicken 67
Passion Fruit Mojito 87
Pecan Crusted Chicken Fingers 38
Pesto Deviled Eggs 24
Pigs in a Blanket 31
Pineapple Cheese Spread 19
Pomegranate Margarita 85
Potato Hummus 25
Praline Pecans 82

R

Raspberry Cosmopolitan 89
Red Hot Chicken Bits 39
Roasted Tomato, Onion & Goat Cheese Frittatini 9

S

Salsa Deviled Eggs 23
Shrimp and Crab Cakes 57
Shrimp Cocktail 61
Shrimp Mold Spread 59
Shrimp with Jalapeno Cheese 60
Skordalia (Greek) 26
Smoked Salmon Triangles 53
So Cheesy Beer & Spinach Dip 16
South African Spicy Potato Noodles 72
Spanikopita 71
Spanish Tomato Toast (Pan con Tomate) 77
Spicy Bean Salsa 73
Spinach Brownies 30
Spinach & Cheddar Whole Wheat Quesadillas 15
Spinach Roll-Ups 25
Spirited Apricot Brie 20
Strawberry Bread 18
Strawberry-Cheese Ball 20
Stuffed Cherry Tomatoes 19
Super Sausage Balls 31
Sweet and Sour Meatballs 47
Sweet Potato Balls 83
Sweet Weiners 80

T

Tempura Avocado with Shrimp 65
Terry's Caribbean Cosmopolitan 89
Tomato and Onion Tart 33
Tostaditas with Gulf Crab 60

V

Valerie's Asian Pasta Salad 63
Valerie's Asian Potstickers 64
Valerie's Fruit Cocktail 88
Veal, Beef, and Pork Meatballs 47
Vietnamese Salad Rolls 55

W

Warm Black Olives 3
White Chocolate Pretzels 81
Wonton Wrapper Appetizers 22
Wrap-and-Roll Basil Pinwheels 24

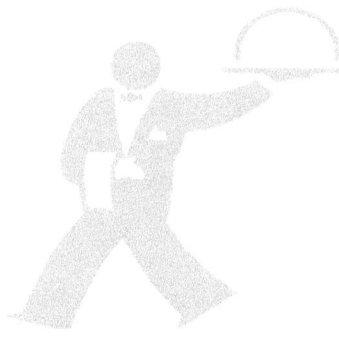

www.ingramcontent.com/pod-product-compliance
Ingram Content Group UK Ltd.
Pitfield, Milton Keynes, MK11 3LW, UK
UKHW051254180426
11947UKWH00020B/1704